Dictionary of
Health Economics

Alan Earl-Slater

RADCLIFFE MEDICAL PRESS

©1999 Alan Earl-Slater

Radcliffe Medical Press Ltd
18 Marcham Road, Abingdon, Oxon OX14 1AA

British Library Cataloguing in Publication Data

A catalogue record for this book is available from the British Library.

ISBN 1 85775 337 2

Typeset by Advance Typesetting Ltd, Oxon
Printed and bound by Biddles Ltd, Guildford and King's Lynn

Preface

Health economics is a rapidly growing discipline. This is due to the increasing interest in finding ways to improve the use of scarce resources that have alternative uses.

This book is very much a reflection of the common terms used in health economics. It is, like the discipline, an important and evolutionary step.

The objectives of this book are to:

- introduce many of the terms used by health economists

- extend the range of terms used in the discipline

- make the terminology accessible and clear

- contribute to the standardisation of the terminology

- improve the understanding of the meaning of the terms.

This book will be useful to the types of people I have taught over the years: doctors, community pharmacists, midwives, public health managers, hospital pharmacists, nurses, pharmaceutical advisers, finance managers, insurance company personnel, practice managers, pharmaceutical company sales executives, staff involved in R & D, government employees, consultants, trainee teachers in health economics, postgraduate and undergraduate students on courses in management, health, policy, social studies and business studies.

How can you use this book? Here are some ideas.

- If you come across a term that may be used in health economics and need clarification of its meaning, refer to this book.

- If you want to learn some of the tools of the trade of health economists, refer to this book.

- If you want to use health economic terminology in your own work, check with this book that you are using the correct term.

- Participate – send me a note if there is a term that you think should be included in the next edition of the book or if you have good examples of a term that a wider audience would appreciate seeing.

I have successfully taught health economics in various places and to various audiences over the years. Examples include St John's Medical School, Bangalore, India; Faculty of Health Sciences, Moi University, Kenya; and at UK universities. I feel very fortunate to have taught health economics to people from over 50 countries in the world. I remain grateful for the wonderful enthusiasm, hospitality and insight that I have received from those that I have taught and worked with. I am grateful to them for encouraging me to write this book.

Alan Earl-Slater
www.2020oxfordpharma.org
March 1999

This book is dedicated to
Elaine, Emmanuela and Maria

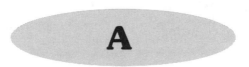

A

Ability to pay

The capability of a person or organisation to pay for a healthcare product. *See* **Willingness to pay**.

Absolute advantage

Occurs when one organisation produces a greater level of goods and services than another from a set of resources, inputs. Table 1 shows two hospitals, A and B, each of which produces two services, cataract operations and hernia repairs, at the same cost. Hospital A can produce 80 cataract operations or 90 hernia repairs. Hospital B can produce 100 hernia repairs or 120 cataract operations. It follows that hospital B has an absolute advantage in both cataract operations and hernia repairs. It can produce more of the two healthcare services. *See* **Comparative advantage; Economies of scale; Economies of scope**.

Table I Absolute advantage

	Hospital A	Hospital B
Hernia repair	80	100
Cataract operations	90	120

Absolute poverty

A situation of destitution, penury or privation such that a person lacks at least one of three basic factors required for survival, namely food, shelter or clothing. It is a state of poverty that is not related to any average or benchmark figure. *See* **Carstairs' index of deprivation; Department of Employment index for planning; Jarman's index of deprivation; Relative poverty; Townsend's index of deprivation**.

Absolute risk

The risk of an event occurring.

Table 2 Absolute risk

	Outcome		Total	Risk of events
	Event occurs	Event does not occur		
New care or exposure	a (1)	b (2)	a + b = 3	X = a/(a + b) = 1/3
Usual care or not exposed	c (3)	d (4)	c + d = 7	Y = c/(c + d) = 3/7
Totals	a + c = 4	b + d = 6	a + b + c + d = 10	

Referring to Table 2, the absolute risk of the event occurring in the new care or exposed group is:

$$ARx = a/(a + b) = X$$

The absolute risk of the event occurring in the usual care or non-exposed group is:

$$ARnotx = c/(c + d) = Y$$

Using data in Table 2 as an example:

$$ARx = 1/(1 + 2) = 1/3 = 0.33$$

which means the absolute risk of the event, e.g. stroke, occurring in the new care or exposed group is 33%.

$$ARnotx = 3/(3 + 4) = 3/7 = 0.49$$

which means the absolute risk of the event, e.g. stroke, occurring in the usual care or non-exposed group is 49%. *See* **Absolute risk reduction; Incidence; Likelihood ratio; Odds; Odds ratio; Relative risk; Relative risk reduction**.

Absolute risk reduction
The difference between the rates of events in two groups. The groups can differ by the care regime they receive or their exposure to a risk factor.

Table 3 Absolute risk reduction

	Outcome			
	Event occurs	Event does not occur	Total	Risk of events
New care or exposure	a (1)	b (2)	a + b = 3	X = a/(a + b) = 1/3
Usual care or not exposed	c (3)	d (4)	c + d = 7	Y = c/(c + d) = 3/7
Totals	a + c = 4	b + d = 6	a + b + c + d = 10	

More generally, then, using the notation in Table 3:

$$ARR = Y - X$$

Suppose the numbers in Table 3 relate to obese patients on current (usual) treatment or on a new treatment with the medication orlistat, in conjunction with a specified hypocaloric diet and exercise programme. Suppose the event is stroke and we are interested to see if the new care regime provides better outcomes than the usual care regime organised by the primary care group. Taking the numbers in Table 3 as an example, we have:

$$ARR = 3/7 - 1/3 = 0.10 \text{ or } (10\%)$$

which means, for instance, the new care programme reduces the chance of stroke by 10% compared to the existing programme. The reciprocal of the ARR is the number needed to treat to achieve a result. *See* **Absolute risk; Likelihood ratio; Number needed to treat; Odds; Odds ratio; Relative risk; Relative risk reduction.**

Accountability
Arises when a person is answerable to another person or organisation for an action or task they have taken or were supposed to have taken. *See* **Due process; Governance; Regulation; Transparency.**

Activities of daily living

Those actions that are considered standard to daily living. Examples include washing oneself, getting in and out of bed, housework, dressing oneself, preparing a meal and eating. The activities that a person can perform and the degree of difficulty that a person experiences can be found by asking the patient to perform certain tasks and recording their ability, or lack of it, in doing these tasks. Activities of daily living (ADL) can also be determined by asking the patient to complete a set of questions relating to the activities. The questions can be graded on a Likert Scale by the degree of difficulty the person has in doing the tasks. An example response to the question 'Can you dress yourself?' could be 1. Not at all; 2. With severe difficulty; 3. With moderate difficulty; 4. With little difficulty; or 5. With no difficulty. The answers can also be determined by asking the patient to complete a visual analogue scale, a continuous line graded from 0 to 100, with 0 reflecting that the person cannot dress themselves and 100 representing that they can dress themselves with no difficulty.

The economic relevance of the ADL is that they can help determine the needs of the patient and therefore what resources would best fit these needs. For example, social and home care may be required rather than healthcare as such. They can also be used to show the impact of healthcare intervention by recording ADL before and after the health intervention. *See* **EuroQol; Health index; Health outcomes measurement pyramid; Health profile; Health status; Index of health-related quality of life; Likert Scale; Nottingham Health Profile; Quality of life; Short-form 36; Surrogate endpoints**.

Adaptive expectations

A conceptual notion about how people make decisions. According to the concept of adaptive expectations, when making forecasts about the future people adapt their expectations on the basis of their past and present ideas, knowledge and experience adjusted in proportion to the size and direction of the error they made in their last decision or forecast. The error term reflects the difference between what actually happened last time and what they expected to happen. In adaptive expectations there is no knowledge of the future: decisions are made in the light of what is known in current and past terms. Therefore when the error term is non-zero adaptive expectations always over- or underestimate the value of an expected variable. People, sick or healthy, may use adaptive expectations. The formula for adaptive expectations can be written as follows:

$$E_t - E_{t-1} = x \, (A_t - E_{t-1})$$

with E_t the expected event in time $_t$, E_{t-1} the expectations at time $_{t-1}$, A_t is what actually happened in time $_t$, and x is the coefficient of adjustment. Notice there is nothing about the future in the formula. *See* **Rational expectations**.

Additive effect

The addition of effects from more than one healthcare intervention. Suppose three interventions are provided: T is the kidney transplant, D the kidney transplant antirejection medicine, E an appropriate patient education video. If T results in t, D in d and E in e and the effects are simply additive, then the final effect of the three interventions is t + d + e. One problem is that each single effect may be of somewhat different importance. Weights can be used to assign the degrees of importance to each effect. *See* **Multiplicative effect**.

Adverse selection

An event in healthcare whereby one party decides not to reveal the full extent of their risk profile to the other party. People at higher risks are more likely to seek health insurance cover but they will not wish to show they are high risks. Some people may be left uninsured as a result of adverse selection: those of low risk who do not bother to take up insurance as the premiums are too high and those of high risk who cannot get insurance as they cannot afford the premiums. *See* **Moral hazard**.

Aggregate demand

The total demand in a market in a particular time period. Suppose two groups of patients, 1 and 2, have the demand schedules D1 and D2 for a product as outlined in Figure 1 respectively. Then, aggregate demand for the product is the sum of D1 and D2, i.e. D3 as shown in Figure 1. *See* **Aggregate supply**; **Demand**.

Aggregate supply

Total supply to a market in a particular time period. Suppose there are only two pharmaceutical companies, 1 and 2, and they have the supply schedules S1 and S2 for non-prescription medication as outlined in Figure 2 respectively. Then the aggregate supply of non-prescription medication is the sum of S1 and S2, i.e. S3 as shown in Figure 2. *See* **Aggregate demand**; **Supply**.

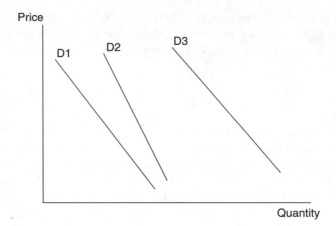

Figure 1 Aggregate demand

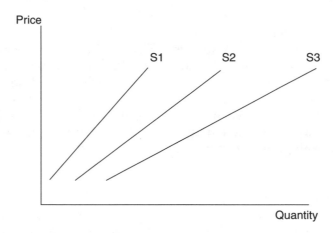

Figure 2 Aggregate supply

Allocative efficiency
A concept in health economics where no improvement is possible in the economy by any redistribution of resources, incentives or rewards in the system. *See* **Efficacy; Efficiency; Pareto optimal; Technical efficiency**.

Alternative hypothesis
A statement that there is a specified relationship or difference between factors under study. For example, a detoxified alcoholic taking the medicine

acamprosate and staying off the alcohol. *See* **Duhem's irrefutability theory;**
Falsificationism; Lakatosian hard-core, protective belt; Null hypothesis.

Analytic perspective

Refers to the viewpoint adopted in an analysis. Examples include the
patient's perspective, the pharmaceutical company perspective, the
prescriber's perspective, the purchaser's perspective, government perspective, a wider society perspective. *See* **Due process; Economic assess-**
ment decision tree; Health measurement pyramid; Value for money
table.

ASTRO-PU

An acronym for Age, Sex, Temporary Resident Originated Prescribing
Unit. The main reason for the calculus is that age and gender affect
prescribing, as may residential status. Adjusting the prescribing data for
these three factors allows more refined comparisons of prescribing over
time and between prescribers. ASTRO-PU is also used in some parts of the
country to help calculate prescribing budgets. In essence, it is a form of
standardisation. Table 4 provides the detail of ASTRO-PU weights. Rather
than just saying that 36 million NHS prescriptions were dispensed in the
Yorkshire Region, the data can be adjusted to reflect Yorkshire's demographic age and gender profile and an adjustment can be made
for the proportion of people classified as being temporarily resident in
Yorkshire.

Table 4 ASTRO-PU weights (1997 version)

Age group (years)	Male: weights	Female: weights
0–4	1.0	0.8
5–14	1.4	1.2
15–24	1.7	2.1
25–34	2.0	2.4
35–44	2.8	3.2
45–54	4.4	5.4
55–64	7.6	7.2
65–74	10.1	9.6
75+	11.8	10.6
Temporary resident	0.5	0.5

See **DDD; General Practice Research Database; PACT; STAR-PU.**

Asymmetric information
A situation whereby parties have different information sets. Hospitals may have greater information about clinical activity than the healthcare purchasers; insured patients may have greater individual information about their behaviour and risks of illness than the insurer; physicians generally have greater information about available healthcare interventions than their patients.

Average benefit
The total benefit divided by the number of people receiving the intervention. *See* **Average cost; Marginal benefit**.

Average cost
The total cost divided by the total quantity. *See* **Average cost pricing; Marginal cost; Total cost**.

Average cost pricing
The practice of setting price equal to the average cost. *See* **Average cost; Break-even diagram; Profit; Threshold point analysis**.

Average fixed cost
Total fixed cost of producing units, divided by the number of units produced. If a pharmaceutical company producing generic products has total fixed costs of £4m per annum and produces 20m drugs per annum, then the average fixed cost is £0.20 (£4 000 000/20 000 000). More generally, the average fixed cost (AFC) is calculated as follows:

$$AFC = \frac{\text{Total fixed cost}}{\text{Quantity}}$$

See **Average total cost; Average variable cost; Fixed cost**.

Average propensity to consume
The rate of total expenditure to total income. If, throughout the year, the patient's total income is £15 000 and they spend £12 000, then their

average propensity to consume is 0.8 (£12 000/£15 000). More generally, the average propensity to consume (APC) is calculated as follows:

$$APC = \frac{Total\ expenditure}{Total\ income}$$

See **Average propensity to save**.

Average propensity to save

The rate of total savings to total income. If, throughout the year, the patient's total income is £15 000 and they spend £12 000 then they save £3000. Their average propensity to save is 0.2 (£3000/£15 000). More generally, the average propensity to save (APS) is calculated as follows:

$$APS = \frac{Total\ savings}{Total\ income}$$

See **Average propensity to consume**.

Average revenue

The total revenue divided by the quantity of units of output. If the health clinic's total revenue is £560 000 per annum and it provides 4500 finished consultant episodes (FCE), its average revenue is £124.44 per FCE (£560 000/4500). The £124.44 is what the health clinic earns on average. See **Demand curve**.

Average total cost

The rate of total cost of producing units divided by the quantity of units produced. The average total cost (ATC) is calculated as follows:

$$ATC = \frac{Total\ costs}{Quantity}$$

See **Average fixed cost; Average variable cost; Total cost**.

Average variable cost

The total variable cost of producing units divided by the number of units produced. More generally, the average variable cost (AVC) is calculated as follows:

$$AVC = \frac{\text{Variable costs}}{\text{Quantity}}$$

See **Average fixed cost; Average total cost; Variable cost.**

Avoided costs

Those costs that have been prevented by taking a course of action. For example, combination treatment with acamprosate calcium in association with counselling of a detoxified alcoholic may help avoid various costs to society: avoiding hospital costs such as dealing with liver cirrhosis; avoiding judicial costs on drunk and disorderly charges; avoiding solicitor's fees when reconciliation occurs rather than separation and divorce.

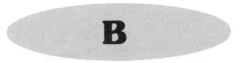

B

Barrier to entry

Anything that deters a product, person, group of people or organisation from entering a market. For example, medicines have to have a market licence before they can come to the market. Barriers to entry are not necessarily detrimental to economic welfare. *See* **Barrier to exit**; **Medicines Control Agency**; **Regulation**.

Barrier to exit

Anything that deters a product, person, group of people or organisation from leaving a market; for example, staff redundancy payments or statutory obligations to supply or fulfil existing contracts. *See* **Barrier to entry**; **Regulation**.

Bilateral monopoly

Occurs in a market when there is only one supplier of the healthcare product and only one purchaser. If, in one city, there is only one hospital and if there is only one effective purchaser, say a primary care group, then this is a bilateral monopoly situation. It may be the case that a single supplier of hospital services (monopolist) will seek to raise prices and lower volumes and quality, whereas the single purchaser (monopsonist) will seek to pay a lower price and receive higher volumes and quality. Unless there are checks and balances influencing the market, the market operators may become complacent and inefficient. *See* **Contestable market**; **Monopoly**; **Monopsony**; **Oligopoly**; **Oligopsony**.

Binary variable

A variable with two possible outcomes. Examples include dead/alive, heads/tails, yes/no, on/off. *See* **Categorical variable**; **Continuous variable**.

Blacklist

A register of prohibited products, people or healthcare units. In 1985 the UK government excluded over 600 medicines from the UK's National Health Service (NHS) reimbursement and in 1997 it produced a list of 60 more products it was seeking to blacklist (not reimburse under the NHS healthcare system). A clinician may have a list of organisations that he will not work for. A healthcare purchaser may have a list of clinics that they will not buy from. A community pharmacy locum may have a list of community pharmacies that she will not work for. A manager may have a list of clinical tests that the consultants will not be allowed to use in the hospital. Who makes the blacklist, on what criteria and with what economic effects are some of the issues to consider. Sometimes the blacklist is called the negative list. *See* **Formulary; Negative list; Regulation.**

Break-even diagram

A diagram which shows the locus of total income and total expenditure. The break-even point occurs where the loci intersect. Figure 3 shows one set of loci. In some cases there may be more than one break-even point.

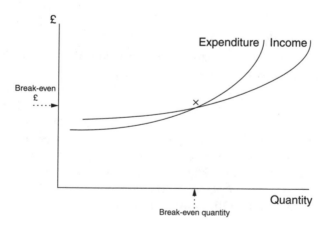

Figure 3 Break-even diagram

Figure 4 shows multiple break-even points. *See* **Profits**.

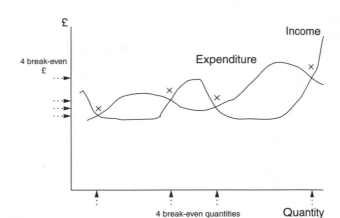

Figure 4 Multiple break-even points

British Medical Journal guidelines for economic evaluations

On 3 August 1996 the *British Medical Journal* (BMJ) published a set of guidelines for economic evaluations. The guidelines are primarily to help BMJ reviewers and the BMJ editorial team determine the quality of economic evaluation papers. However, the guidelines also help authors and researchers in their design and writing up of economic evaluations and in the interpretation of studies. The guidelines are set out in the form of 35 questions reproduced in Table 5. Thirty-five questions may seem substantial but they are not comprehensive, nor does each question necessarily have equal weight or importance.

For more detail on the guidelines read the relevant BMJ article. *See* **Compliance cost assessment; Economic assessment decision tree; Guidance on Good Practice in the Conduct of Economic Evaluations of Medicines; National Institute of Clinical Excellence; Regulatory Impact Analysis**.

Table 5 *British Medical Journal* guidelines for economic evaluations

1 The research question is stated.
2 The economic importance of the research question is stated.
3 The viewpoint(s) of the analysis are clearly stated and justified.
4 The rationale for choosing the alternative programmes or interventions compared is stated.
5 The alternatives being compared are clearly described.
6 The form of economic evaluation used is stated.
7 The choice of form of economic evaluation is justified in relation to the questions addressed.
8 The source(s) of effectiveness estimates used are stated.
9 Details of the design and results of effectiveness study are given (if based on a single study).
10 Details of the method of synthesis or meta-analysis of estimates are given (if based on an overview of a number of effectiveness studies).
11 The primary outcome measure(s) for the economic evaluation are clearly stated.
12 Methods to value health states and other benefits are stated.
13 Details of the subjects from whom valuations were obtained are given.
14 Productivity changes (if included) are reported separately.
15 The relevance of productivity changes to the study question is discussed.
16 Quantities of resources are reported separately from their unit costs.
17 Methods for the estimation of quantities and unit costs are described.
18 Currency and price data are recorded.
19 Details of currency or price adjustments for inflation or currency conversion are given.
20 Details of any model used are given.
21 The choice of model used and any key parameters on which it is based are justified.
22 Time horizon of costs and benefits is stated.
23 The discount rate(s) is stated.
24 The choice of the rate(s) is justified.
25 An explanation is given if costs or benefits are not discounted.
26 Details of statistical tests and confidence intervals are given for stochastic data.
27 The approach to sensitivity analysis is given.
28 The choice of variables for sensitivity analysis is justified.
29 The range over which the variables are varied are justified.
30 Relevant alternatives are compared.
31 Incremental analysis is reported.
32 Major outcomes are presented in a disaggregated as well as aggregated form.
33 The answer to the study question is given.
34 Conclusions follow from the data reported.
35 Conclusions are accompanied by the appropriate caveats.

Budget locus

The combinations of goods or services that a person or organisation can buy with their set of funds. Figure 5 shows linear and non-linear budget loci. The importance of a budget locus is that it depicts the maximum combinations of goods and services that can be bought by the person or organisation with a given set of funds. At points below the budget locus the person or organisation is not spending all their available funds. At points above the budget locus the person or organisation is exceeding their available funds. The slope of the budget locus depends on the relative prices of the goods or services. The budget loci may not be continuous.

Suppose two services are available, S1 and S2, then the slope of the budget locus is the marginal rate of substitution between service S1 and service S2. A steeper slope suggests a higher marginal rate of substitution. A more moderate or gentle slope suggests a lower marginal rate of substitution.

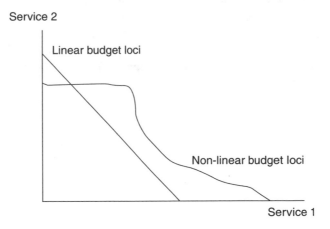

Figure 5 Budget loci

In Figure 6 the linear budget line will move from BL1 to BL2 if the *price* of product A falls. In Figure 6, BL2 will shift to BL3 if the purchaser's *income* falls.

Budget loci can be used in association with indifference curves to help establish the best possible combinations of goods and services to buy. *See* **Indifference curve**.

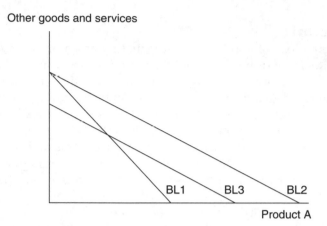

Figure 6 Budget loci movement

Buyers' market

Exists when there are more goods or services available for sale than there are buyers for them in the market. It follows that in these conditions of excess supply, the buyers have the upper hand in negotiations. Buyers can pay lower prices, receive higher quality or greater quantity of the goods and services. *See* **Equilibrium; Excess supply; Sellers' market.**

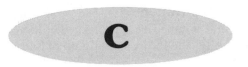

C

Capital:labour ratio

The proportion of capital employed to labour employed to produce a unit of output. Different healthcare professionals have different capital:labour ratios. For example, primary care doctors and nurses have relatively low capital:labour ratios, whereas hospital surgeons and radiographers have higher capital:labour ratios.

Capitation

A technique of paying or allocating resources based on the number of people in a group. For example, primary care doctors can receive capitation-based budgets with which to buy some or all of their population's healthcare services based on the number of people on the doctor's register. Weights can be attached to the capitation formula to allow for differences within a group. For example, in the calculus more weight may be given to older patients than to younger patients as older patients generally use more healthcare goods and services than do younger patients. *See* **ASTRO-PU; DDD; Per capita; STAR-PU**.

Cardinal utility

If utility can be measured in cardinal terms then statements can be made about one person's utility compared to another person's or how much utility one person gets from different levels of consumption. For example, if utility is cardinal then statements such as the following can be made: Mrs Reid receives twice as much utility from taking a 'once-a-day' medicine than from taking another medicine three times a day; Mrs Reid receives three times as much utility from consuming medicine A than Mrs Smyth receives from consuming medicine A. Therefore if utility is cardinal, the degree of differences in utility can be expressed and held to have meaning. *See* **Cost–utility analysis; Ordinal utility; Priority setting; Utility**.

Carstair's index of deprivation

A single number that is taken to represent the degree of deprivation of people in a community. The index is made up of four components:

1 unemployed male residents over 16 years of age as a proportion of all economically active male residents over 16 years of age in the community;

2 the number of people in households with one or more persons per room as a proportion of all residents in households in the community;

3 the number of residents in households without a car as a proportion of all residents in households in the community;

4 the number of persons in households with an economically active head of the household categorised in social class IV or V as a proportion of all residents in households in the community.

Each component in the Carstair's index of deprivation has the same weight. The four components are then standardised by a Z-score and the index is simply the sum of the standardised scores. The greater the Carstair's index number, the greater the deprivation of the community. *See* **Absolute poverty; Department of Employment index for planning; Index number; Jarman's index of deprivation; Poverty trap; Relative poverty; Townsend's index of deprivation; Z-score.**

Categorical variable

A variable that has a finite number of possible outcomes but no logical order. Examples include race, gender, marital status, residential status, blood group. *See* **Binary variable; Continuous variable.**

Certainty equivalent

An amount of money that a person would require with certainty, to make them indifferent between the certain sum and the uncertain sum. For example, a person may be indifferent between receiving £100 with certainty or £1000 with a probability of 5%. *See* **Indifference curve.**

Ceteris paribus

The Latin term for 'other things remain equal'. It is often used in economic modelling. The reason for using *ceteris paribus* as an assumption is to tease out the effects of a specific factor on another, when everything else is assumed to remain the same. Its validity depends on how much is known about the market and the importance of other factors that may actually change and influence events. *See* **Sensitivity analysis**.

Clinical governance
A new framework through which NHS organisations are accountable for continuously improving the quality of their services. *See* **Accountability; Corporate governance; Due process; Governance; Regulation; Transparency**.

Commission for Health Improvement
A new national body in the NHS with the remit of supporting and overseeing the quality of clinical governance and clinical services. *See* **Clinical governance**.

Committee on Safety of Medicines
A UK committee composed of around 30 independent experts with secretariat support, meeting every fortnight, with the responsibility of assessing an application for a product licence and making recommendations to the UK ministers of health (politicians) as to whether, and on what terms, the product should be licensed in the UK. *See* **Medicines Control Agency**.

Comparative advantage
A situation where people are employed in areas in which they perform relatively better than others. Comparative advantage implies that people should specialise in whatever they have the advantage in. Table 6 shows two hospitals, A and B, each of which is able to provide two services: cataract operations and hernia repairs.

Table 6 Comparative advantage

	Hospital A	Hospital B
Cataract operations	80	100
Hernia repairs	90	120

Hospital A can provide 80 cataract operations or 90 hernia repairs. Hospital B can provide 100 cataract operations or 120 hernia repairs. Hospital

B can produce more of each from the set of resources: it therefore has an absolute advantage in both services.

Mathematically the cataract-to-hernias ratios are $80/90 = 0.88$ for hospital A and $100/120 = 0.83$ for hospital B. Hospital A has a comparative advantage in cataract services and should therefore provide these as it has the highest ratio ($0.88 > 0.83$). Again, mathematically, the hernias-to-cataract ratios are $90/80 = 1.125$ for hospital A and $120/100 = 1.2$ for hospital B. Therefore hospital B has a comparative advantage in hernia operations and should provide hernia operations as it has the highest ratio ($1.2 > 1.125$). See **Absolute advantage; Economies of scale; Economies of scope**.

Compensating principle

The notion that those who gain from a decision could compensate those who lose. It does not mean that the winners do actually compensate the losers for their loss. Further, it does not mean that the economy would overall be better off from the decision to compensate.

Suppose a change in the economy causes everyone's well-being to improve; then unambiguously, people are better off than before as the economy and everyone in it have improved. Suppose a change in the economy causes only some people to be better off but no one worse off; then, on balance, the economy has again improved.

Imagine a third scenario: some people's well-being is improved but others are worse off. In this scenario, is the economy better off than before? One way to answer that question is to use the compensating principle: the people whose welfare has increased could compensate those whose welfare has worsened. It is not necessary that the transfer takes place, but if it could and if no one was left worse off than before and at least one person is better off than before, then the economy has improved in net welfare terms. See **Externalities; Pareto improvement; Pigovian subsidy; Pigovian tax; Potential Pareto improvement; Slutsky decomposition; Welfare**.

Complementary demand for goods or services

Goods or services that have the characteristic that their use or consumption is interdependent. For example, nurses and hospital beds may be in complementary demand whereby a demand for more beds means a demand for more nurses. Goods or services that are complements in demand can be determined mathematically by using the cross price elasticity of demand. See **Complementary supply of goods or services; Cross price elasticity of demand; Indifference curve; Substitutes**.

Complementary supply of goods and services

Goods or services that have the characteristic that their supply is inter-dependent. Whether or not goods or services are complements in supply can be determined mathematically by using the cross price elasticity of supply. *See* **Complementary demand for goods or services; Cross price elasticity of supply; Substitutes**.

Compliance

The extent to which patients adhere to the advice given by their healthcare provider. For example, obese patients may go on a programme of a mildly hypocaloric diet with 30% of calories as fat, the medicine orlistat and multivitamin supplements. The economic angle is that if patients do not fully comply with the appropriate care programme, the medicine on its own may have little of the desired effect and therefore be a waste of resources. Sometimes compliance is called concordance. *See* **Effectiveness; Efficacy; Efficiency**.

Compliance Cost Assessment (UK government)

In 1985 the UK government introduced a framework for assessing its proposed policies. The audit framework and instrument still exists and is called the Compliance Cost Assessment (CCA). The CCA was part of the enthusiastic drive towards evidence-based decision making in the government. The UK's Department of Trade and Industry declared that:

> A CCA is a structured appraisal that all government departments must prepare when evaluating policy proposals likely to affect business. Its purpose is to inform Ministers and officials of the likely costs to business of complying with new or amended regulations so that compliance costs can be assessed, and unnecessary burdens to business identified well before a decision is taken on whether or not to go ahead with the proposals.

The CCAs are to:

> ... provide scope for improving the balance between costs and benefits ... (the) procedure is intended to ensure that all proposals for new regulations meet the government's other policy objectives (and) have been properly considered for the requirements they will place

on business and that, taking all policy considerations into account, the new regulation is justified.

In 1985 the UK government set up an Enterprise and Deregulation Unit (renamed in May 1997 as the Better Regulation Unit). In addition to its general government departmental business, each government department was obliged to carry out three processes:

1 to provide a systematic *ad-hoc* account of the impact on business of existing regulations;

2 to identify possible burdens of all new regulatory proposals in six-monthly 'forward looks';

3 to carry out a CCA in relation to all proposals.

CCA audits were to provide the details shown in Table 7.

Table 7 CCA audit details

1	An outline of the purpose of the measure and a brief description of how it would remedy a specific problem.
2	An outline of the wider benefits of the measure and quantify them where possible.
3	A statement of the business sectors or types of businesses likely to be affected and an estimate of the number of businesses involved.
4	A description of any significant features of the business sectors.
5	A summary of the total estimated compliance cost of the measure for a 'typical' business in the sectors principally affected.
6	Illustrate what percentage of turnover of the 'typical business' is represented by these compliance costs.
7	If using a 'typical business' may give a misleading impression, then illustrate the impact on different types of notional businesses likely to be affected.
8	A summary of the total estimated compliance costs for all specific sectors or types of businesses likely to be affected.
9	Where the cost of the measure would be phased over more than one year, a statement of the number of years and the year in which the costs would start.
10	An indication of how any additional costs arising from the measure might affect the competitive position of UK-based business.
11	Demonstrate the extent of consultation, identify the sources and describe any consultations with business.
12	Declare the arrangements for monitoring and reviewing the impact of the policy.
13	If a different approach would have achieved the objectives of the proposed measures at lower cost, give an explanation of why this was or should be rejected.
14	Finally, all preliminary and published CCAs should give a contact point for enquiries and comments.

The CCA audit is concerned with the costs, direct, indirect and intangible, and with the benefits. It is also concerned with consultation with interested or affected parties and with the opportunity cost of a decision.

The CCA audit is concerned with:

1 a spatial aspect, i.e. *who* would get *what*;

2 a temporal dimension, *when*;

3 an impact or distribution dimension on *how* the parties identified would get the costs and benefits; and

4 an opportunity cost consideration.

It is interesting to note that CCAs were rarely used in respect of healthcare policy under the Conservative government (1979–97) although that government was responsible for CCAs and major healthcare reform when in power. *See* **British Medical Journal guidelines for economic evaluations; Guidance on Good Practice in the Conduct of Economic Evaluations of Medicines; Opportunity cost; Regulation; Regulatory Impact Assessment.**

Concentration ratio
A measure of market share. *See* **Market power; Market share**.

Conjoint analysis
Methods of establishing the factors that influence a person's demand for goods and services. Five steps in conjoint analysis are: identifying factors to be included in the study; assigning values to these; presenting realistic scenarios for the person to choose between; recording their preferences; collating and analysing the results. Sometimes called vignette analysis. *See* **Ability to pay; Derive demand; Standard gamble; Time trade-off; Willingness to pay**.

Consumer's surplus
The difference between the value a consumer places on a healthcare product and the amount they actually pay. Suppose a community service made a product available at £1200 but nobody bought it; at a price of £1100 one person would buy one unit. At £800 the person would buy two units

and at £500 the person would buy three units. Suppose the supplier decides to supply three units at £500 each. Then at £500 the person buys three units and there is no excess supply or demand. But the person was willing to pay £1100 for one unit, £800 for the second unit and £500 for the third. It follows that because the person actually pays only £500 for each of three units she secures consumer's surplus to the value of £900 ((£1100 – £500) + (£800 – £500) + (£500 – £500)).

Consumer's surplus can be represented by the amount above the market price that people are willing to pay compared to what they actually pay.

More generally, total consumer's surplus is the sum of individual consumer's surplus on each unit: area xyz as shown in Figure 7. Suppliers can try to reduce consumer's surplus by engaging in price discrimination. *See* **Price discrimination; Producer's surplus**.

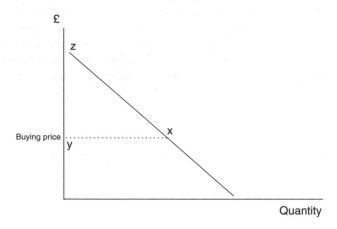

Figure 7 Consumer's surplus

Contestable market
A contestable market is one in which there are no barriers to entry or exit. This freedom of entry and exit acts as a spur to a firm's efficiency. So, even if there is only one firm in the market it may still be efficient if the market is perfectly contestable. *See* **Barrier to entry; Barrier to exit**.

Contingent valuation
One way of determining how much a person is willing to pay for certain healthcare goods or services. For example, how much a person values a treatment option will be contingent on a variety of factors. Examples of

factors that some patients have considered when valuing a healthcare intervention include: what results they expect to see; when the results are expected; the probabilities of achieving the results; their degree of trust of healthcare professionals; their knowledge of their own past and others' experiences; how unbearable their present condition is; what after-care service is required; who is going to pay for the intervention; and when the intervention would actually be obtained. *See* **Conjoint analysis; Willingness to pay.**

Continuous variable
A variable that can differ by an infinitesimally small amount. Examples include cholesterol level, body mass, temperature, height and weight. *See* **Binary variable; Categorical variable.**

Contributory benefit
Occurs when a benefit is awarded to a person or organisation if and only if they have made the necessary contributions to the finance of such. *See* **Means testing; Non-contributory benefit.**

Copayment
An amount paid by the patient partly covering the cost of the healthcare provided to them. Sometimes called user charges. *See* **User charges.**

Corporate governance
A new framework through which NHS organisations are accountable for the standards in conducting corporate business including meeting statutory financial duties. *See* **Accountability; Clinical governance; Due process; Governance; Regulation; Transparency.**

Cost (form of cost)
There are various forms of cost: total, fixed, semifixed, variable, average, marginal and opportunity cost. *See* **Average cost; Cost (where costs fall); Fixed cost; Marginal cost; Opportunity cost; Semifixed cost; Total cost; Variable cost.**

Cost (where costs fall)
Costs can fall in three areas: direct costs, indirect costs and intangible costs. *See* **Cost (form of cost); Direct cost; Indirect cost; Intangible cost.**

Cost analysis
A type of economic assessment that portrays the costs of an intervention. *See* **Cost (form of cost); Cost (where costs fall); Economic assessment decision tree**.

Cost–benefit analysis
A type of economic assessment that considers the costs and effects of at least two alternative courses of action, where costs and benefits are measured in money terms. Cost–benefit analysis does not assume *a priori* that the outcomes from the intervention are worthwhile. It can be used when there are multiple outcomes provided they can be recast in money terms. There are serious and inherent difficulties in calculating outcomes in money terms: for example, how does one accurately calculate in money terms the value of lives saved in the treatment of ventricular arrhythmia? One possible procedure is to determine what people are willing to pay for certain sets of outcomes and use these results as the relevant monetary units. *See* **Cost-effectiveness analysis; Cost-minimisation analysis; Cost–utility analysis; Economic assessment decision tree; Incremental analysis; Marginal analysis; Value for money table**.

Cost centre
A unit in an organisation whereby all its activities are identified and costed. The identification and measurement of costs for the unit can then be used to signal what the unit has to charge or receive to be covering its costs. Establishment of cost centres can help provide useful information, education and incentives for the unit's staff and for the wider organisation on the costs the centre incurs. *See* **Virement**.

Cost-effectiveness analysis
A type of economic assessment that considers the costs and effects of at least two types of possible intervention where the effects are different, but measured in natural units. Examples of natural units are: cholesterol level, visual acuity, body mass, lumbar flexion, blood pressure, number of inoculations, incidence of the ill health condition, prevalence of the condition, the number of lives saved and mortality rates.

   For example, a hospital operation A costs £1350 for the electro-physiology stimulation in treatment of ventricular arrhythmias. Suppose that the hospital intervention saves the lives of eight out of ten patients.

The alternative healthcare intervention is a course of medicine B at a cost of £750 per course. Suppose the intervention with medicine is successful in six out of ten patients. On the basis of the evidence of costs and effects, which option provides better value for money, A or B? One way to make a decision on these data is to calculate the cost per unit effect. In the example above, the cost per unit effect is the cost per life-year saved. A course of hospital electrophysiology stimulation costs £1687.50 (£13 500/8) per life saved. A course of medication in a primary care intervention regime costs £1250 (£7500/6) per life saved. On the basis of this evidence, intervention in primary care is more cost-effective than hospital electrophysiology stimulation in the treatment of ventricular arrhythmias.

As there are usually multiple outcomes from healthcare intervention, the difficulty is how to reconcile any portfolio of outcomes. One solution would be to recalculate the portfolio of outcomes into a single common unit of measurement: an index number. Another possible solution is for a decision to be made, and made explicit, on what is the most important outcome in the portfolio and just use that as the unit of outcome measurement. So in the example above, the lives saved is probably the most important end-point or outcome in the treatment of ventricular arrhythmia. An intermediate position is to assign weights to the various outcomes in the portfolio and calculate a weighted basket of outcomes. *See* **Cost–benefit analysis; Cost-minimisation analysis; Cost–utility analysis; Economic assessment decision tree; Incremental analysis; Index number; Marginal analysis; Value for money table**.

Cost-of-burden study

An assessment of the full burden of a disease in terms of what costs are involved, when they occur and where (e.g. an anti-Alzheimer's disease medicine may delay patients with Alzheimer's disease entering residential care homes). *See* **Cost (form of cost); Cost (where costs fall); Value for money table**.

Cost-minimisation analysis

A type of economic assessment that considers the costs and effects of at least two types of intervention where the effects are found to be, or can be assumed to be, the same or not significantly different. The medicines acamprosate and bromocriptine are alternative adjuncts to levodopa in a detoxified alcoholic's maintenance of abstinence from alcohol care programme. One published randomised control clinical trial found the outcomes to be essentially the same. On this basis, the appropriate type of analysis to undertake is a cost-minimisation analysis. With similarity of outcomes, if treatment regimen A costs more than B, the doctor would opt for treatment regime B; that is, she would minimise the costs of achieving the same outcome by going for choice B. This is cost-minimisation analysis: comparing the costs of more than one course of possible intervention when the outcomes from each intervention are alike. Strictly speaking, the outcomes have to be of the same magnitude and distribution between the possible interventions.

Multiple or single outcomes from healthcare intervention are captured. The only proviso is that the package of outcomes from each intervention is found to be the same or not significantly different or that the packages of outcomes can be safely assumed to be alike. Thus, the actual units of measurement are irrelevant to cost-minimisation analysis. *See* **Cost–benefit analysis; Cost-effectiveness analysis; Cost–utility analysis; Economic assessment decision tree; Incremental analysis; Marginal analysis; Value for money table**.

Cost–utility analysis

A type of economic assessment that considers the costs and effects of at least two types of possible healthcare interventions where the effects are not the same but are measured in units of utility or satisfaction. As with cost–benefit analysis, cost–utility analysis can be used when there are multiple effects of healthcare intervention. One way to determine the outcomes in utility terms is to use the concept of the quality-adjusted life-year (QALY). For example, suppose a hospital operation A costs £1350 for the electrophysiology stimulation in treatment of ventricular arrhythmia and that the hospital intervention provides 800 QALYs. The alternative healthcare intervention is a course of medicine B at a cost of £750 per course which provides 600 QALYs. Is intervention A better value for money than intervention B? One way to make a decision on these data is to calculate the cost per QALY gained. A course of hospital electrophysiology stimulation costs £1.69 (£1350/800) per QALY gained. Primary care intervention with medicine costs £1.25 (£750/600) per QALY. On the basis of this evidence and calculus, intervention with medication in primary care is more cost-effective than hospital electrophysiology stimulation in the treatment of ventricular arrhythmia. The impact of healthcare intervention in terms of utility can be determined by using, for example, quality of life questionnaires or satisfaction reviews. *See* **Cardinal utility; Cost–benefit analysis; Cost-effectiveness analysis; Cost-minimisation analysis; Economic assessment decision tree; Healthy years equivalent; Incremental analysis;**

Marginal analysis; Marginal utility; Ordinal utility; QALY; Value for money table.

Cross price elasticity of demand

The change in demand for one product in response to changes in the price of another. For example, the change in demand for intracavernosal injections in response to the change in the price of oral medication sildenafil for patients with male erectile dysfunction. The cross price elasticity of demand (CP_{ed}) formula is as follows:

$$CP_{ed} = \frac{\% \text{ change in demand of A}}{\% \text{ change in price of B}}$$

See Complementary demand for goods and services; Complementary supply of goods and services; Cross price elasticity of supply; Own price elasticity of demand; Substitutes.

Cross price elasticity of supply

The change in supply of one product in response to changes in the price of another. For example, the change in supply of one anaesthetic product as a result of changes in the price of another. The cross price elasticity of supply (CP_{es}) formula is as follows:

$$CP_{es} = \frac{\% \text{ change in supply of A}}{\% \text{ change in price of B}}$$

See Complementary demand for goods and services; Complementary supply of goods and services; Cross price elasticity of demand; Own price elasticity of supply; Substitutes.

Cross subsidisation

The act of using profits from one activity to subsidise another part of the business, which is inefficient or unprofitable. *See* Cost centre; Economic rent; Profit; Virement.

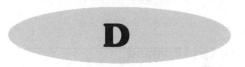

DDD

DDD is an acronym for defined daily dose. The World Health Organisation (WHO) publishes a reference manual on the DDDs of most prescription medicines. The DDD is said to reflect the typical average adult maintenance dose for that medicine per day.

Table 8 Some examples of DDDs

Medicine	DDD
Amoxycillin	1 g
Atenolol	75 mg
Bendrofluazide	2.5 mg
Cimetidine	800 mg
Diclofenac	100 mg
Digoxin	0.25 mg
Frusemide	40 mg
Ibuprofen	1.2 g
Nifedipine	30 mg
Paracetamol	3 g
Prednisolone	10 mg
Propranolol	160 mg
Ranitidine	300 mg
Temazepam	20 mg
Terfenadine	120 mg

Calculations by DDD help standardise prescribing data over time and between practices. DDDs also allow international comparisons of prescribing. DDDs are not perfect benchmarks as:

1 some medicines cannot be converted into DDDs, e.g. vaccines, some dermatologicals;

2 some of the WHO calculations are based on hospital prescribing which may not be comparable with prescribing in the primary care setting;

3 local practice may differ from the WHO's DDD catalogue.

See **ASTRO-PU; General Practice Research Database; PACT; STAR-PU**.

Decision tree

An analytical framework representing choices available, outcomes and probabilities of achieving those outcomes. Suppose the patient has a choice between two alternative courses of action: treatment regime A or treatment regime B. If she chooses regime A then she may secure outcome '1' with a probability of X or outcome '2' with a probability of 1–X. If, however, she chooses regime B then she may secure outcome '3' with a probability of Y or outcome '4' with a probability of 1–Y. Figure 8 displays this detail in a decision tree format. The choice actually made depends on the data associated with the outcomes and their probabilities: that is, the expected values of each option. In general, the best option is the one with the highest expected outcome.

Decision trees can be used to share knowledge, encourage debate and improve decision making. They can also show what data are required to make a decision and reveal the difficulties of getting those data; they can also be constructed to deceive rather than enlighten. *See* **Economic assessment decision tree; Value for money table**.

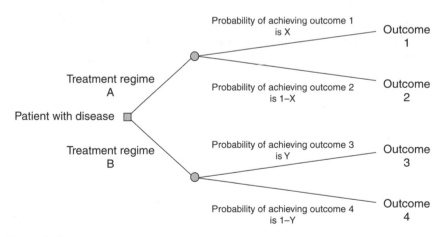

Figure 8 Decision tree

Declining balance technique

A method of discounting assets at declining rates over a period of years. For example, if a magnetic resonance imaging machine is bought at £1m, a declining balance technique may use a 25% discount for the first year, 20% for year 2, 15% for year 3, 10% for year 4 (Table 9). The declining balance technique is useful when assets depreciate highly in their first few years and then have lower depreciation rates over the remaining period.

Table 9 Declining balance technique for magnetic resonance imaging equipment

	Value	Discount Factor	Book value
Year 0	£1m		£1m
Year 1		25%	£750 000
Year 2		20%	£600 000
Year 3		15%	£510 000
Year 4		10%	£459 000

See **Discounting; Straight line depreciation**.

Demand
A request for a healthcare product. *See* **Demand curve; Derived demand; Need**.

Demand curve
A locus of quantities of healthcare goods and services that the healthcare purchaser will buy at different possible prices. Figure 9 gives a simple linear example. A distinction is to be made between shifts *in* (*along*) the demand

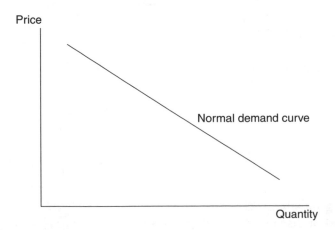

Figure 9 Demand curve

curve (which can be caused by changes in the price of the product) and shifts *of* the demand curve (which can be caused by a change in the consumer's real income; a change in the price of a substitute product; a change in the price of a complementary product; a change in preferences or a change in taxation). *See* **Demand; Giffen good or service; Merit good or service; Normal good or service; Public good or service; Supply curve.**

Demand function
A relationship, sometimes expressed mathematically, between the demand for a healthcare product and all the factors that are said to influence the demand. Influencing factors include: the price of the healthcare product; the price of substitutes; the price of complementary goods or services; the income of the purchaser; insurance coverage and copayments; taxation; individual tastes and preferences; and market regulation. *See* **Demand; Demand curve.**

Department of Employment index for planning
A single number that is said to represent the degree of deprivation of people in a community. The index is made up of six components:

1 unemployed male residents over 16 years of age as a proportion of all economically active residents over 16 years of age in the community;

2 the number of people in households with one or more persons per room as a proportion of all residents in households in the community;

3 the number of households where a pensioner lives alone as a proportion of all households in the community;

4 the number of households where a single parent lives with their offspring as a proportion of all households in the community;

5 the number of residents born in the New Commonwealth as a percentage of all residents in the community;

6 the number of households lacking exclusive use of inside toilet and bath or shower as a proportion of all households in the community.

The calculation of the index is as follows. First, calculate the data for the six elements (e.g. by census survey). Second, take the natural logarithm of components 1, 2, 4, 5 and 6 (not of component 3, notice). Third, calculate the Z-scores of the logarithms of 1, 2, 4, 5, 6 and the Z-score of component 3.

Fourth, apply weights to the resulting data (components 1, 3, 4 have weights of 2 units each, components 2, 5, 6 have weights of 1 unit each). Fifth, add up the numbers to reveal a single index number. The final resulting number is the Department of Employment index for planning.

The greater the index number, the greater the deprivation. Whether the components are valid reflectors of deprivation and whether the method of calculation yields unbiased results is debatable. *See* **Absolute poverty; Carstair's index of deprivation; Index number; Jarman's index of deprivation; Relative poverty; Townsend's index of deprivation**.

Derive demand

The demand for a healthcare product is derived from the demand for the outcomes of that product or service, i.e. improvements in health status or life expectancy. The healthcare goods and services are vehicles for achieving the outcomes. For example, a patient's demand for a medicine is derived, generally, not from the medicine itself but from the benefits the medicine is expected to give her. So, a patient with chronic rheumatoid arthritis may demand an antirheumatic medicine to help ease her plight. *See* **Demand; Need**.

Direct benefit

Direct benefits associated with a healthcare intervention include improvements in the patient's clinical, physical, psychological, mental, social or spiritual well-being. For example, medicines for the treatment of rheumatoid arthritis can yield benefits to patients such as lowering the incidence and severity of joint pain and increasing the patient's grip strength. *See* **Direct cost; Health measurement pyramid; Indirect benefit; Indirect cost; Intangible benefit; Intangible cost; Outcome**.

Direct cost

A cost associated with a healthcare intervention such as clinical investigation cost, laboratory fees, healthcare professional fees and expenses, medication costs, administration and management costs. *See* **Cost (where costs fall); Direct benefit; Indirect cost; Intangible cost**.

Discounting
Two definitions of discounting are:

1 the reduction in the list price for a healthcare product to yield an actual transaction price;

2 reducing future incomes and expenditures to reflect the fact that the value of £1 today is generally higher than £1 in the future.

See **Discount rate**.

Discount rate
A figure used to transform future costs or benefits into present-day values. Two questions are whether the same discount rate is used over time; and whether benefits are discounted at the same rate(s) as costs.

For example, in cancer care, the patient's quality of life drops under chemotherapy intervention and may rise once the treatment has finished.

Should it only be the costs and benefits to patients that are discounted? For example, suppose a new medicine increases the self-caring ability of an elderly man with Parkinson's disease. This medicine will reduce the burden on the carer, his middle-aged daughter. Do the benefits to the middle-aged daughter need to be considered in the calculus? *See* **Declining balance technique; Discounting; Straight line depreciation**.

Disjointed incrementalism
Where decisions are made as the problem evolves through time. *See* **Accountability; Adaptive expectations; Decision tree; Due process; Rational expectations; Transparency**.

Dual labour market hypothesis
The idea that there are two segments to the labour market: a primary segment and a secondary segment. In the primary segment the main characteristics of the jobs are: relatively high wages, good working conditions, stability in employment, opportunities for progress and career advancement, equity and due process in the rules, rewards and engagement of employees. In the secondary segment, the main characteristics of the jobs are: relatively low wages, poor working conditions, no stability in employment, few opportunities for progress or career advancement,

inequities and little due process in the rules, rewards and engagement of employees.

Due process
Occurs when a decision maker states explicitly what their decision is, how they came to it, what the benefits will be, at what cost and what resources (e.g. staff and equipment) will be required. *See* **Accountability; Transparency**.

Duhem's irrefutability theory
Is that no hypothesis can be comprehensively falsified or refuted, as any particular hypothesis always has a series of auxiliary conditions or underlying hypotheses, so that no one can ever be sure of the exact location of any refutation. Thus, refutation is not definite.

If the results of a randomised clinical trial between a new medication and current best practice suggest the new medicine is more cost-effective than current best practice, then under Duhem's irrefutability theory one cannot say without reservation that the new medicine is more cost-effective than current best practice. *See* **Alternative hypothesis; Falsificationism; Lakatosian hard-core, protective belt; Null hypothesis; Systematic review**.

Duopoly
A situation where there are two suppliers of goods or services in a market; for example, two hospitals serving one primary care group. *See* **Duopsony; Imperfect competition; Monopoly; Monopsony; Oligopoly; Oligopsony; Perfect competition**.

Duopsony
A situation where there are two buyers of goods or services in a market. *See* **Duopoly; Monopoly; Monopsony; Oligopoly; Oligopsony; Perfect competition**.

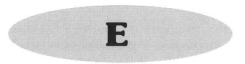

Economic assessment decision tree

A pictorial representation of different methods of economic assessment
available. The first stage in the decision tree asks whether or not costs and
outcomes of healthcare interventions are being considered. The second
stage asks whether or not different possible interventions are compared.

Figure 10 shows the economic assessment decision tree. This can be used
for a variety of purposes: determine what has been done as opposed to
what is said to be done; establish what should be done; ascertain what needs
to be done; reveal the gaps in the evidence; display differences between
various forms of assessment; signal the similarities between methods of
assessment. *See* **Decision tree; Economics; Value for money table**.

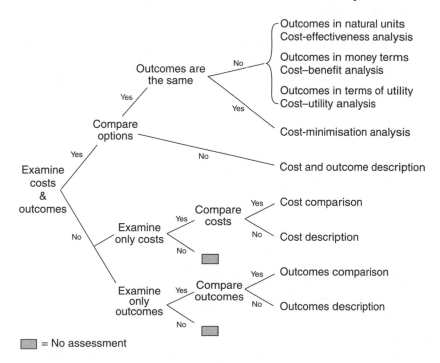

Figure 10 Economic assessment decision tree

Economic rent

The amount of money paid over and above what is actually necessary to keep that factor of production (e.g. staff) in that work. For example, if a community pharmacist earns £38 000 per annum but would continue to work for only £30 000, she is receiving economic rent of £8000 per annum. *See* **Transfer earnings.**

Economics

The study of how people and organisations make use of scarce resources that have alternative uses, and the rewards from their use.

The discipline of economics can be split in various ways. One distinction is between micro economics (concerned with the individual person or organisation) and macro economics (concerned with aggregates of people or organisations). Another distinction is between positive economics (objective) and normative economics (subjective). *See* **Macro economics; Micro economics; Normative economics; Positive economics.**

Economies of scale

The relationship between costs and output. Increasing economies of scale occur when unit costs fall as output rises. Constant economies of scale occur when unit costs do not change as output changes. Decreasing economies of scale occur when unit costs rise as output rises. *See* **Economies of scope; Natural monopoly.**

Economies of scope

The comparison between the costs of one firm doing two activities compared to the cost of two firms each doing one of the activities. Economies of scope arise when the cost of one firm doing two activities is less than the cost of two firms each doing one of the activities.

Mathematically, economies of scope can be written as:

$$C_{f1} (X_1, X_2) \leq C_{f2} (X_1, 0) + C_{f3} (0, X_2)$$

where C_{f1}, C_{f2} and C_{f3} are firms 1, 2 and 3 costs respectively; X_1 is product 1 and X_2 product 2. *See* **Economies of scale.**

Effectiveness

The degree to which a healthcare intervention works in practice. *See* **Efficacy; Randomised control trial; Systematic review.**

Efficacy

The degree to which a healthcare intervention does what it was intended to do under ideal conditions. Thus, randomised control clinical trials, if construed as ideal conditions, may yield evidence of the intervention's efficacy. *See* **Effectiveness; Randomised control trial**.

Efficiency

An expression of the relationship between resource use, processes and outcomes. *See* **Effectiveness; Efficacy; Production possibility curve; Stochastic frontier analysis**.

Elasticity

A measure of the responsiveness of one factor to changes in another. *See* **Cross price elasticity of demand; Cross price elasticity of supply; Elasticity of substitution; Income elasticity of demand; Own price elasticity of demand; Own price elasticity of supply**.

Elasticity of demand

The responsiveness of demand to changes in factors that could affect demand. *See* **Cross price elasticity of demand; Demand function; Elasticity of substitution; Income elasticity of demand; Own price elasticity of demand; Own price elasticity of supply**.

Elasticity of substitution

A measure of the ease of switching between substitute products; for example, the ease in switching between anti-migraine medicines. Other examples include the ease of switching between anti-arthritis medications or in switching between acid suppressant proton pump inhibitors. Beyond medicines the term can relate to the degree of ease in switching patients between hospitals, switching between consultants or switching more generally between care programmes. *See* **Cross price elasticity of demand; Cross price elasticity of supply; Elasticity**.

Elasticity of supply

The responsiveness of supply to changes in factors that could affect supply. *See* **Elasticity of substitution; Income elasticity of demand; Own price elasticity of demand; Own price elasticity of supply; Supply**.

Equilibrium

A market is said to be in equilibrium when demand matches supply and there are no underlying market forces likely to change the situation. The forces for change directly and equivalently match the forces against change. *See* **General equilibrium**; **Partial equilibrium analysis**.

Equity

Relates to fairness or justice. The concept of equity has long been a source of dispute in society due to its subjective and moral overtones. One way into equity debates is to make a distinction between two forms of equity: horizontal equity and vertical equity. Horizontal equity is the equal treatment of equals. Vertical equity is the unequal treatment of unequals.

Various ways to interpret horizontal equity exist. At a general level it relates to the equal treatment of equals but more specifically one could argue for: people with equal clinical need to receive equal clinical treatment; equality of access for equal need; equality of resource use for equal expected health gain; equality of per capita funding for equal need. Whatever area is considered, the principle is the same: horizontal equity is the equal treatment of equals.

A vertical equity argument is that those patients with different clinical needs are treated differently in the system: the unequal treatment of unequals. Vertical equity can relate to people, services or products. Suppose a hospital has two types of possible purchasers for hip replacements and the purchasers differ in the size of their budget: a primary care group and a private health insurer. Should the hospital set up different types of contracts for the purchasers, i.e. should it use the principle of vertical equity in contract setting? *See* **Efficiency**.

Equity–efficiency trade-off

An equity–efficiency trade-off is said to exist when equity is inversely associated with efficiency. If an equity–efficiency trade-off exists, then a rise in equity is accompanied by a fall in efficiency and a fall in equity is accompanied by a rise in efficiency. *See* **Efficiency**; **Equity**; **Trade-off**.

EuroQol

A health status measurement instrument that aims to allow comparison of health status between people of different countries with the same disease or between people with different diseases. The aim is to produce an internationally standardised, valid, reliable and feasible measurement instrument that is not disease specific. EuroQol produces an indication of a person's actual health status (e.g. by asking the patient) or hypothetical valuation of health status (e.g. by asking people how they rate certain possible or hypothetical health states).

Table 10 shows the five dimensions of health in the EuroQol: mobility, self-care, usual activities, pain/discomfort and an anxiety/depression dimension. Each dimension has three elements. This therefore produces a maximum of 243 ($3 \times 3 \times 3 \times 3 \times 3 = 3^5$) possible descriptions of health status.

Table 10 EuroQol

A Mobility
1 No problems in walking about
2 Some problems in walking about
3 Confined to bed

B Self-care
1 No problems with self-care
2 Some problems washing or dressing
3 Unable to wash or dress self

C Usual activities
1 No problems performing usual activities (e.g. work, study, housework, family or leisure)
2 Some problems with performing usual activities
3 Unable to perform usual activities

D Pain/discomfort
1 No pain or discomfort
2 Moderate pain or discomfort
3 Extreme pain or discomfort

E Anxiety/depression
1 Not anxious or depressed
2 Moderately anxious or depressed
3 Extremely anxious or depressed

For example, a EuroQol result of 12223 means a person is considered to have no problems walking about; some problems washing or dressing; some problems performing usual activities; has moderate pain or discomfort; and is extremely anxious or depressed.

More generally, one has to consider: the internal consistency of the dimensions; whether there is any overlap between the five dimensions; and how differences can be reconciled. What methods can be used to combine the results of the five elements to reveal a single index number? Visual analogue scales have been used where the person is asked to complete answers to the five dimensions above and then place a mark on a visual analogue scale as to their perception of their health status. Another issue is how to compare different people's results in order to help resource allocation. Is 12323 of the same value as 13212? With 243 possible health states, how can the results be compared?

A EuroQol Group is working on resolving difficulties with the measurement instrument and strengthening its beneficial aspects (e.g. it helps describe health states). The EuroQol instrument has been used in areas such as cardiovascular disease, cosmetic surgery, diabetes, leukaemia, orthopaedics, urology and road accident victims. *See* **Activities of daily living; Health measurement pyramid; Health profile; Health status; Index of health-related quality of life; Nottingham Health Profile; Quality of life; Short-Form 36; Sickness Impact Profile**.

Excess demand
A situation where there is more demand for a product than there is supply. Under certain conditions where excess demand exists, the price of the product will rise until the demand matches the supply. Those who cannot afford or will not pay the new higher price are effectively priced out of the market: this reduces the total amount of the product demanded. The price is raised until the amount of demand matches the amount of supply to the point where no excess demand or supply exists. *See* **Demand; Equilibrium; Excess supply; Sellers' market; Supply**.

Excess supply
A situation where there is more supply of a product than there is demand. Under certain conditions where excess supply exists, the price will fall until supply matches the demand. Those who cannot or will not supply at the new lower price are effectively priced out of the market: this reduces the total amount of the product supplied in the market. The price falls until the amount of demand matches the amount of supply to the point where no excess supply and no excess demand exists. *See* **Buyers' market; Demand; Equilibrium; Excess demand; Supply**.

Expected utility theory
The collection of techniques for combining the utility of an event and the probability of the event. The results can show which course of action has the best possible expected utility. *See* **Decision tree; Utility**.

External benefits

Arise when one activity generates benefits to a party that is not subject to the bargain struck. Suppose a patient has a hip replacement. An external benefit of this would be the effect that intervention has on her carer to reduce the amount or type of care they now have to give. For example, before the operation the patient may have been getting help with her weekly shopping and housekeeping from her family or a care agency. Once she has had the operation she usually no longer needs such assistance. It can be argued that the existence of external benefits are not fully acknowledged in healthcare purchasers' priority setting where they only look at the patient and not the patient's more holistic circumstances. It can also be argued that where there are external benefits of healthcare intervention then the parties who stand to benefit, e.g. the welfare or care agencies, could help the patient get the intervention sooner rather than later, by making a financial contribution to the cost of the intervention. This suggests that a more holistic approach to purchasing and prioritising healthcare may improve the use of resources. *See* **External costs; Externalities; Pigovian subsidy.**

External costs

Arise when one activity generates costs to a third party that is not subject to the bargain. If a patient is on HRT, then an external cost of this would be the effect that therapy has on the woman's family. For example, the family may experience the consequences of her suffering side effects such as mood swings and tiredness. It can be argued that the existence of external costs are not fully covered in healthcare purchasers' priority setting where they only look at the patient and not the patient's more holistic circumstances. It can also be argued that where there are external costs of healthcare intervention then the parties who stand to bear these costs could provide information so that the intervention could come at a different time or in a different way. As with external benefits, the existence of external costs can suggest that a more holistic approach to purchasing and prioritising healthcare may improve the use of resources. *See* **External benefits; Externalities; Pigovian tax.**

Externalities

Spillovers from people's activities which affect a third party in a positive or negative way. A positive externality is a benefit to a third party and a negative externality is a cost to a third party as a result of other parties' activities. If a hospital landscapes its grounds then this will benefit the householders living nearby. If an elderly person receives a hip replacement then her husband will also benefit when she can engage in more activities of daily living herself. Externalities can be seen where the social costs and benefits of an action do not match the private costs and benefits of the action. *See* **External benefits; External costs; Pigovian subsidy; Pigovian tax.**

External validity of results

The extent to which the results of a study are valid in another place or at another time. Otherwise called generalisability, transferability or applicability of study results. *See* **Efficacy; Efficiency; Internal validity of results; Systematic review.**

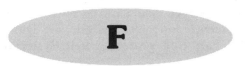

F

False-negative rate

The proportion of negative test results in patients with the disease. In Table 11 the false negatives are assigned to the quadrant with the letter 'c' and the false-negative rate (FNR) is 'c/(a + c)'. Using the numbers in Table 11, the FNR = 30/(10 + 30) = 0.75

Table 11 False-negative rates

	True condition of the person tested		
Test result	Has the adverse medical condition	Does not have the adverse medical condition	Total
Positive	a (10)	b (20)	a + b (30)
Negative	c (30)	d (40)	c + d (70)
Total	a + c (40)	b + d (60)	a + b + c + d (100)

See **False-positive rate; Sensitivity; Specificity; True-negative rate; True-positive rate.**

False-positive rate

The proportion of positive test results in patients without the disease. In Table 11, the false positives are assigned to the quadrant with the letter 'b' and the false-positive rate (FPR) is 'b/(b + d)'. Using the numbers in Table 11, the FPR = 20/(20 + 40) = 0.33. *See* **False-negative rate; Sensitivity; Specificity; True-negative rate; True-positive rate.**

Falsificationism

The belief that the validity of a theory depends on whether or not it is falsified by empirical evidence. Simple falsification is where the theory is discarded if it is falsified by one empirical test. Sustained falsification is where a theory is discarded when it is falsified by more than one empirical test. Theories are provisionally accepted until they are falsified. Falsification-ism is used in areas such as systematic reviews, evidence-based decision making, medical science and meta-analysis. *See* **Duhem's irrefutability theory; Lakatosian hard-core, protective belt; Systematic review.**

Fisher diagram
Shows a model of consumer's preference for consumption in two time periods. In any time period the consumer can consume or invest certain amounts. Figure 11 shows an example of a person with income Y1 in period 1, consuming C1 in period 1. In this period an amount Y1 – C1 has not been spent. Then, in period 2 the consumer has income Y2 and savings of Y1 – C1 and can consume at point C2. In period 2 they achieve utility Z. By not consuming all their income in period 1, they can increase their utility in period 2. *See* **Budget locus; Discounting; Indifference curve; Marginal propensity to consume; Marginal propensity to save.**

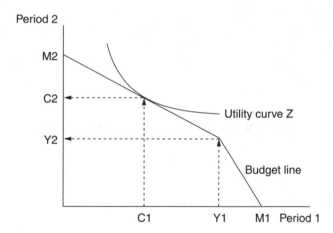

Figure 11 Fisher diagram

Fisher's index
Is an index number calculated from two other index numbers. It is the geometric mean of the Laspeyre index and the Paasche index. As the Laspeyre index overstates movement in the data series and the Paasche index understates movement, the Fisher index is said to be a closer representation of reality. If L represents the Laspeyre index and

P represents the Paasche index, then Fisher's index, F, is calculated as follows:

$$F = \sqrt{(L \times P)}$$

So, for example, if L = 3.5 and P = 2.4, then the Fisher's index = 2.9. *See* **Index number; Laspeyre index; Paasche index**.

Fixed costs
Those costs that do not vary with activity levels. Therefore fixed costs have to be paid irrespective of activity levels. The higher the fixed costs, the greater the barrier to entry to a market. *See* **Barrier to entry; Cost (form of cost); Cost (where costs fall); Marginal costs; Semifixed costs; Total costs; Variable costs**.

Formulary
A list of goods or services that meet certain criteria of acceptance. Usually considered as those goods and services that are eligible for use or those that will be reimbursed by the healthcare financier. For example, most hospitals have a restricted list of medicines that can be used in their setting. A formulary is one way of making explicit the selection of medicines to be used by the health professionals. Underlying the idea of a medicines formulary are concerns about making good use of resources, controlling medicine activity and therefore, to an extent, medicine expenditure. The criteria to get on a formulary, the reasons for delisting, who designed the formulary and the scope of the formulary are some of the issues to consider. Sometimes called a positive list. *See* **Blacklist; Negative list; Positive list**.

Free goods and services
In economic terms, free goods and services have two essential characteristics: first, there is no price for them and second, there are no property rights on ownership or use. Air, wind, sunshine, rain and snow may be considered free goods and services. If a hospital consultant receives a set of clinical instruments as a 'free gift' from a medical instruments company then this is not a free good as someone somewhere has incurred costs in making and delivering such. *See* **Merit good or service; Public good or service**.

Free rider problem

Occurs when those who do not pay for the healthcare product cannot be prevented from consuming the product. Other examples include pacifists being protected by national defence programmes, liberalists being protected by the judiciary and legal system. *See* **Externalities**.

Future years of life lost

A measure of loss as a result of premature mortality. It is measured by the difference between the population life expectancy and the patient's actual age at death.

So if a man dies at 63 from cardiac arrest and the average life expectancy of men aged 63 is 12 years, then the future years of life lost is 12. If the base period for life expectancy is taken to be at birth, then the population of males at birth may have a life expectancy of 78 years. Therefore, on this base, the future years of life lost to the cardiac patient is 15 (78 – 63). It is important therefore to know the basis of the life expectancy in the calculus. *See* **Life expectancy**.

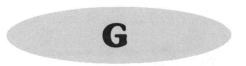

G

Gambler's fallacy
The idea that if a chance event has not happened for some time, it is bound to occur soon.

General equilibrium
A situation in the economy where all markets clear, there being no excess demand or supply in any market. *See* **Equilibrium; Excess demand; Excess supply; Macro economics; Partial equilibrium analysis**.

General Practice Research Database
This is a database of NHS primary care prescribing. It covers 525 practices, 3.4m patients and prescribing histories from 1987. Uniquely, it provides patient specific detail, e.g. diagnosis, what the drug was actually prescribed for. It provides information on product volume, variety, number of patients and diagnosis. Strengths of using the General Practice Research Database (GPRD) are: the data already exists; immediate access to licence holders; there is no need to recruit patients or GPs into any particular study; there is no interference with doctor or patient decisions; the database is flexible (i.e. a variety of studies and methods of analysis can be used on the database); the UK's Office of National Statistics quality checks and provides the database. Furthermore, whilst databases such as PACT can yield information on volume and cost, GPRD can be used to help establish effectiveness, appropriateness, switching between medicines, patient numbers involved, what the drug is prescribed for, some outcomes, and lead into value for money analysis. *See* **ASTRO-PU; DDD; PACT; STAR-PU; Transparency**.

Geographic information system
A system for capturing, storing, checking, manipulating and displaying data which is spatially referenced. For example, it can be used to identify the number of prescriptions written by primary care groups or dispensed

in different localities. Computer software packages are available to help perform the work.

Giffen good or service

One for which the demand varies directly with price. If the price of a Giffen good or service rises, demand rises. If the price of a Giffen good or service falls, demand falls. Figure 12 shows the picture. *See* **Income effect; Inferior good or service; Merit good or service; Normal good or service; Public good or service; Slutsky decomposition; Substitution effect**.

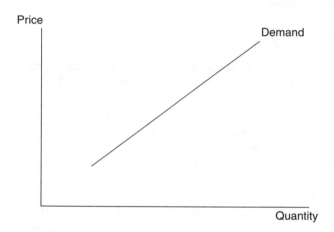

Figure 12 Giffen good or service

Gini coefficient

The Gini coefficient (G) is an estimation of the amount of inequality of a factor across a population. A Gini coefficient of 0 suggests no inequality whereas a Gini coefficient of 1 suggests only one person or organisation has all the factor. The lower the G, the lower the inequality. One factor commonly used is income and so the Gini coefficient can measure the inequality of income in a population. Mathematically, the Gini coefficient is written as follows:

$$G = \frac{\text{Area between Lorenz curve and 45\% line}}{\text{Total area below 45\% line}}$$

Alternatively, by referring to Figure 13, this can be written as:

$$G = \frac{\text{Area A}}{\text{Area A} + \text{Area B}}$$

In Figure 13 the horizontal axis shows the percentage of the population in the economy and the vertical axis shows the percentage of income in the economy. So at point X, on the actual income distribution line, 40% of the population have 10% of the income. At point Y, 80% of the population have 40% of the income. At point Z, on the 45° equity line, 50% of the population would have 50% of the income.

In reference to Figure 13, the Gini coefficient is measured by area A divided by areas A and B. The greater the inequality of income, the greater the area A. The greater the area A, the larger the Gini coefficient. Put slightly differently, the higher the Gini coefficient, the greater the inequality.

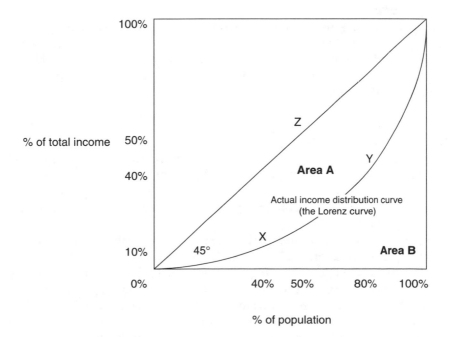

Figure 13 Gini coefficient calculated from the Lorenz curve diagram

Global health index

A single figure which is said to represent the entire health status of a person at a particular period of time. *See* **EuroQol; Health; Health gain; Health index; Health measurement pyramid; Health profile; Health status; Index of health-related quality of life; Nottingham Health Profile; Sickness Impact Profile**.

Gold standard

An ideal measure, technique, or result against which all other measures, techniques and results can be compared. *See* **Randomised control trial; Systematic review; Yardstick pricing**.

Governance

Another term for regulation. *See* **Clinical governance; Corporate governance; Regulation**.

Grey literature

Publications not generally available, not published in large quantities, not readily distributed and not generally indexed in public domain reference systems. For example, pharmaceutical companies have a substantial body of grey literature on file with respect to clinical trials on their products. *See* **Systematic review**.

Gross domestic product

A measure of total economic activity in an economy. It is the sum of all incomes, corporate and personal, earned in the economy from the production of goods and services. One use of the gross domestic product (GDP) is to consider how much the economy spends on healthcare goods and services as a proportion of GDP.

In 1995, total public and private expenditure on healthcare was, at market prices, on average, 7.9% of GDP for members of the Organisation for Economic Co-operation and Development (OECD). For the UK the total healthcare expenditure as a proportion of GDP at market prices was 6.9%. The two polar extremes were Greece, at 5.5%, and the US at 14.5%.

Total healthcare expenditure as a proportion of GDP is often used to argue that if a country is below average this implies its healthcare is under-funded. Yet there is actually no correct ratio of total healthcare expenditure as a proportion of GDP, even if some think there is and others want to believe there is. *See* **Gross national product**.

Gross national product
A measure of total economic activity of residents in an economy. It is the sum of all incomes, corporate and personal, before provision for capital amortisation, earned by residents in an economy, including the residents' income from overseas enterprise and property, but excluding the corresponding income in the economy earned by non-residents. *See* **Gross domestic product**.

Guidance on Good Practice in the Conduct of Economic Evaluations of Medicines (UK)
On 20 May 1994 a Joint Working Party of the Joint Working Group of the UK Department of Health and a pharmaceutical companies' representative body in the UK, the Association of the British Pharmaceutical Industry (ABPI), produced the non-compulsory *Guidance on Good Practice in the Conduct of Economic Evaluations of Medicines* (Table 12). The working party suggested that the government and the pharmaceutical industry want to see a value for money health service in which economic evaluation plays a role in purchasing and prescribing medicines for human consumption.

Table 12

---

1 The question being addressed by the study, including the demographic characteristics of the target population group, should be identified and be set out at the start of the report of the study.
2 The conceptual and practical reasons for choosing the comparator should be set out and justified in the report of the study.
3 The treatment paths of the options being compared should be identified, fully described, placed in context of overall treatments and reported. Decision analytic techniques can be helpful in this regard.
4 The perspective of the study should ideally be societal, identifying the impact on all parts of society, including patients, the NHS, other providers of care and the wider economy. However, costs and outcomes should be reported in a disaggregated way so that the recipients of costs and outcomes can be identified. Attention should be drawn to any significant distributional implications. Indirect costs should normally be included in a societal perspective although care should be taken to avoid any double-counting and the results should be reported including and excluding these costs.
5 The study should use a recognised technique. These include cost-minimisation analysis (CMA), cost-effectiveness analysis (CEA), cost–utility analysis (CUA) and

(continued overleaf)

(Table 12 *continued*)
cost–benefit analysis (CBA). Any one of these could be appropriate according to the purpose of the study. The report of the study should include justification of the technique chosen.

6 In choosing the method of data capture and analysis, the use of one of, or a combination of, prospective or retrospective randomised control clinical trials, meta-analysis, observational data and modelling should be considered. The reasons for the choice of method and, where relevant, for the choice of trials should be reported.

7 Assessment of the question should include determining and reporting what additional benefit is being provided at what extra cost using incremental analysis of costs and outcomes.

8 Outcome measures should be identified and the basis for their selection reported. Where CUA is used, proven generic measures of quality of life are preferred.

9 All relevant costs should be identified, collated and reported. Physical units of resources used should be collected and reported separately from information about the costs of the resources. Costs should reflect full opportunity cost, including the cost of capital and administrative and support costs where relevant. Average costs data are often acceptable as a proxy for long-run marginal cost.

10 Discounting should be undertaken on two different bases:
   A all cost and outcomes discounted at the prevailing rate recommended by the Treasury, currently 6% per annum;
   B all costs and monetary outcomes discounted at the Treasury rate, currently 6% per annum, but non-monetary outcomes not discounted. Both sets of results should be reported. The physical units and values of costs and outcomes prior to discounting should also be reported.

11 Sensitivity analysis should be conducted and reported. The sensitivity of the results to all uncertainty in the study should be explored. This should involve the use of confidence intervals and/or ranges for key parameters, as appropriate. The ranges and choice of parameters to vary should be justified.

12 Comparisons with results from other studies should be handled with care. Particular attention should be paid to differences in methodology (such as the treatment of indirect costs) or differences in circumstances (such as different population groups).

The guidelines are available to be used on a voluntary basis. *See* **British Medical Journal guidelines for economic evaluations; Compliance cost assessment; Discounting; Economic assessment decision tree; National Institute of Clinical Excellence; Regulatory impact analysis**.

Guttman Scale

A health status measurement scale that contains a series of hierarchical statements about an issue where respondents are asked to identify an affirmative point on the scale and that if they agree with any item on the scale this implies that they agree with all items that have lower value on the scale. An individual score is the rank of the most extreme statement the person endorses. Guttman Scales have been used for the physical function of patients who have had a stroke or a hip replacement and for the impact of arthritis on patients' ability to feed, bathe, clothe themselves or walk. *See* **Health gain; Health measurement pyramid; Health needs; Index of health-related quality of life; Likert Scale; QALY; Visual analogue scale.**

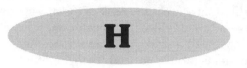

H

Halo effect
Occurs when a person's performance is overrated. *See* **Hawthorne effect**; **Health gain; Hello-goodbye effect**.

Hawthorne effect
The very fact that people are under study, observation or investigation can have an effect on the way they behave and on the results of the study. A Hawthorne effect can either be positive or negative or a mixture of both (and therefore not necessarily detected).

The Hawthorne effect was first noted in the results of studies of Elton Mayo and others at the Western Electric Plant, Hawthorne, USA in the 1920s and 1930s. They studied the effects on productivity of improving lighting in one part of a factory and not changing the lighting in another part. It was found that productivity improved in both parts of the factory. The improved productivity in the part of the factory where lighting did not change was attributed to what is now called the Hawthorne effect.

Health
In 1948 the World Health Organisation defined health as 'A state of complete physical, mental, and social well-being and not merely the absence of disease or infirmity'. It suggests, therefore, that health is not just determined by healthcare. *See* **Health status**.

Health action zones
A new policy initiative from the UK government aiming to promote innovative approaches to public health and community care.

Health authority
Organisations in the UK National Health Service which have been established to manage healthcare delivery for patients in a specific geographic area.

The government announced in December 1997 that some of the key tasks of health authorities would be:

1 assessing the health needs of the local population;

2 drawing up a strategy for meeting those needs, in the form of a health improvement programme;

3 deciding on the range and location of healthcare services;

4 determining local standards and targets to drive quality and efficiency;

5 supporting the development of primary care groups;

6 allocating resources to primary care groups;

7 holding to account primary care groups in its area.

See **Health action zones; Health improvement programme; National Health Service trusts; Primary care group; Regulation.**

Health economics
The study of how people and organisations make use of scarce resources and the rewards achieved in terms of health (quantity and quality of life). *See* **Economic assessment decision tree; Economics; Health measurement pyramid; Value for money table.**

Health gain
The addition to health status that someone has or can have from an intervention. In many cases healthcare can improve the health status of the person. In order to have some indication of the magnitude of the health gain, one needs to measure the person's health status before and after the intervention. There are instruments available to measure health but whether they capture all the relevant dimensions of the person's health remains debatable. The concept of health gain is of interest as one basis for allocating resources to those who can gain the most. As health is not just determined by healthcare, allocating healthcare resources according to who could gain the most from them is not always the most efficient way to improve someone's health status or make the best use of scarce resources. *See* **Health; Health index; Health measurement pyramid; Health profile; Index of health-related quality of life; QALY.**

Health improvement programme

A new policy initiative from the UK government to encourage the development of action programmes aiming to improve health and healthcare locally. Led by the health authority, health improvement programmes (HImPs) will involve NHS trusts, primary care groups and other primary care professionals working in partnership with local authorities and engaging other local interests. *See* **Health authority; Health action zones; Health gain; National Health Service trusts; Primary care group**.

Health index

A single number which is said to represent the health status of a person. *See* **Health measurement pyramid; Health profile; Index of health-related quality of life; Index number**.

Health measurement pyramid

A conceptual device in the shape of a two-dimensional pyramid. On the base of the pyramid are six elements of health status, higher up the pyramid are health profiles and at the top of the pyramid are health indices. Figure 14 gives an example.

Keeping the base elements separate leads to a health *profile*. Adding the base elements together leads to a health *index*. It may be argued that reading along the base of the health measurement pyramid from left to right, the elements become more subjective whereas reading from right to left, the elements become less subjective or more scientific.

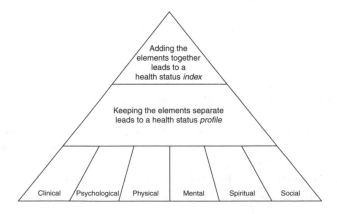

Figure 14 Health measurement pyramid

The pyramid can be used for a variety of purposes: to compare measures; to determine what is and what is not in a measurement.

Two issues to consider are first, not all health profiles or health indices include every one of the six basic components of health; second, in some indices and profiles that do include the same elements in their composition, they may have used different questionnaires, tests or surveys to elicit the measure. *See* **Health; Health index; Health profile; Health status**.

Health production function
A mathematical formula which expresses the outputs of various different inputs to health. *See* **Health**.

Health profile
A collection of information, in the form of a portfolio, that is said to represent the health status of the person surveyed. *See* **Health index; Health measurement pyramid; Health status**.

Health status
The state of well-being of a person. An individual's well-being depends, amongst other things, on their residential conditions, diet, education, income, family conditions, occupation, personality, spirituality, religious beliefs, personal security, community sanitation, wider environmental factors such as relatively clean air, a lack of noise, pollution and access to healthcare facilities. Therefore healthcare is only one factor affecting people's health status. *See* **Health; Health gain; Health index; Health measurement pyramid; Health profile; Index of health-related quality of life**.

Healthy worker effect
The situation whereby people in gainful employment have lower mortality or morbidity rates than other groups of people. The healthy worker effect occurs because employers choose healthier people for jobs and sicker people tend to leave employment. The healthy worker effect can influence the generalisability and validity of clinical trials and priorities in healthcare resource allocation decisions. *See* **Health status**.

Healthy years equivalent
Reflects the number of years that could be spent in perfect health compared to the number of years spent in imperfect health. For example,

10 years of perfect health may be considered as equivalent to 16 years with angina. *See* **QALY; Standard gamble; Time trade-off**.

Hello-goodbye effect
Part of the psychodynamics of some people whereby they initially present themselves in the worst possible light to become eligible for treatment and then, after treatment, present themselves in the best possible light in an attempt to signal substantial gain in their condition. If uncorrected, the health gain of the patient will be overestimated. The hello-goodbye effect is a serious threat to the validity of clinical studies, meta-analysis and policy making. *See* **Health gain; Health index; Health measurement pyramid; Health status; Systematic review**.

Heterogeneous product
A product which is in some way different from similar, but not identical, goods and services. For example, over 40 types of portable blood test equipment are available in the market today. *See* **Homogeneous product**.

Historic cost
The initial purchase price of an asset.

Homogeneous product
A product which is not different, or not perceived to be different, from another product. This means some standardisation, or perception of standardisation, of the goods or services in question. *See* **Heterogeneous product**.

Horizontal equity
The equal treatment of equals. *See* **Equity; Vertical equity**.

Horizontal integration
Where one establishment joins another at the same stage of production of a product. Suppose two firms produce synthetic porous medical swabs: if the two firms unite this is an example of horizontal integration. Horizontal integration may increase market power and reduce consumer choice. It can also enable structural reform in an industry, reduce excess capacity,

improve research and development efforts and limit duplication. *See* **Vertical integration**.

Hotel costs
Those costs incurred in a healthcare unit which are not clinical costs; food, heating, ventilation and linen are some examples.

Human capital
The skills, knowledge and orientation of an individual. It can be improved by investment in education, training or experience.

Human capital method
A technique of estimating the indirect costs of sickness or premature death. It is normally calculated as earnings lost as a result of a person's sickness or premature death. *See* **Cost (form of cost); Human capital; Indirect cost; Life expectancy**.

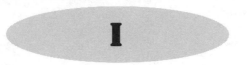

I

Imperfect competition

An economic concept of a market whereby all firms are not price takers, so that at least one firm's behaviour can affect the market price. The market is usually characterised by at least one of the following: heterogeneous health-care goods or services, imperfect information about market conditions, barriers to entry or barriers to exit from the market. *See* **Heterogeneous product**; **Imperfect oligopoly**; **Monopoly**; **Perfect competition**; **Perfect oligopoly**.

Imperfect markets

Occur when there is a departure from the perfect market as defined by economists. For example, social costs may depart from social benefits, private costs of a healthcare intervention may depart from private benefits. Allocative and technical efficiency cannot be achieved in imperfect markets. *See* **Efficiency**.

Imperfect oligopoly

An economic concept of a market whereby there are a small number of firms in the market each producing differentiated goods or services. Dimensions of differentiation may be price, aftersales service, quality, brand image and loyalty, advertising, clinical amenity, non-clinical amenity, speed of access to the healthcare service. *See* **Imperfect competition**; **Monopoly**; **Perfect competition**; **Perfect oligopoly**; **Price competition**.

Incidence rate

The incidence rate (IR) is an estimate of the risk of developing a disease. Mathematically, the IR is the number of new cases of a disease occurring, divided by the number of people exposed to the risk of developing the disease during that time period:

$$IR = \frac{\text{Number of new cases}}{\text{Population exposed}} \times 1000$$

See **Prevalence rate**.

Income–consumption curve

A locus of points that show how consumption changes when income changes, holding prices constant. It can be determined by the use of indifference maps and budget lines. Figure 15 gives an example.

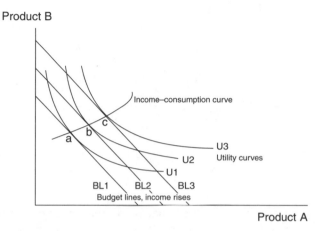

Figure 15 Income–consumption curve

Suppose the consumer uses their income to buy two products, A and B. If income rises then the budget lines move out, in parallel, from BL1 to BL2 or BL3 and utility rises from U1 to U2 or U3 respectively. The income–consumption curve is the locus of points where the utility curves U1, U2, U3 are tangential to the budget lines BL1, BL2, BL3 respectively, i.e. at points a, b and c. *See* **Budget locus; Income effect; Indifference curve; Price–consumption curve; Slutsky decomposition; Substitution effect; Utility**.

Income effect

When the price of a product changes this has two effects on demand: an income effect and a substitution effect. The income effect is the change in demand for a product due to a change in real income when the price of the product changes (Figure 16). Starting at X, the price of product A falls so budget line moves to BL2, utility to U2 and consumer to point Y. Plot BL3 parallel to BL2 (showing the change in real income) and the income effect then is measured by the horizontal difference between points ZY. For example, if the price of a medicine falls by 50%, from the same budget the

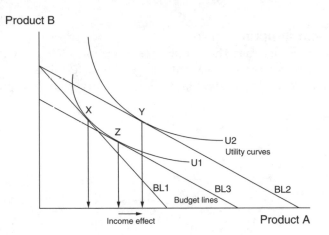

Figure 16 Income effect

primary care group can buy more of that medicine or other goods and services. In effect, a fall in price means that the spending power of the budget has risen (equivalent to a rise in real income).

The income effect need not be of the same magnitude or even in the same direction as the substitution effect. The net effect of a price change is found by adding the income effect to the substitution effect. The net effect on demand resulting from a price change can be lower demand (negative net effect), no change in demand (neutral) or increased demand (positive). *See* **Slutsky decomposition; Substitution effect.**

Income elasticity of demand

A measure of the change in demand for a product as a result of changes in the income of the purchaser. Mathematically, the income elasticity of demand (I_{ed}) is calculated as follows:

$$I_{ed} = \frac{\% \text{ change in demand}}{\% \text{ change in income}}$$

An I_{ed} greater than 1 suggests an elastic demand with respect to income. I_{ed} less than 1 suggests inelastic demand with respect to income. The greater the I_{ed}, the greater the responsiveness of demand to changes in income. *See* **Elasticity; Own price elasticity of demand.**

Incremental analysis

A calculation that determines the difference in costs of two options, divided by the difference in outcomes of the two options.

For example, two healthcare options for treating detoxified alcoholics include medicines A or B. The programmes also include psychosocial counselling and assessment. Suppose the care path with A costs £1400 per patient per year and with B it costs £1000 per patient per year. Suppose the main outcome of interest is the number of abstinent days and the programme with medicine A yields 240 abstinent days while the programme with medicine B yields 200 abstinent days. The incremental analysis result is £10 per abstinent day gained (i.e. (£1400 – £1000)/(240 – 200)). This suggests that programme with medicine A costs an additional £10 per abstinent day gained compared to programme B.

Mathematically, the incremental analysis (IA) calculation is as follows:

$$IA = \frac{\text{Cost of A} - \text{Cost of B}}{\text{Outcomes from A} - \text{Outcomes from B}}$$

See **Marginal analysis; Programme budgeting; Zero-based budgeting.**

Index number

A single number which aims to represent a change in a collection of numbers. There are a variety of ways to construct index numbers and they have a variety of uses. The most famous index number is the retail price index, a measure of the change in the retail prices of a notional basket of goods and services over some time period. Because not all goods and services in the basket may be of equal importance, greater weights can be applied to those considered more important to the average person's expenditure than the others in the basket. See **Fisher's index; Laspeyre index; Paasche index.**

Index of health-related quality of life

A summary measure of a person's quality of life developed by Professor R Rosser and colleagues. The index has three dimensions: disability, discomfort and distress. Within each dimension there are different states of health: eight states of disability, five states of discomfort and five states of distress.

Disability

D1 No physical disability; perfectly mobile and physically active; able to perform all self-care and role functions.

D2 Slight social disability, e.g. having a slight cold. No limitations with physical ability, self-care or mobility but some role functions slightly impaired by social disability.

D3 Slight physical disability. Able to get around house and community, but unable to perform heavy physical tasks. Role functions slightly limited by physical disability. Able to perform all self-care activities.

D4 Able to get around house and do lighter physical work. Some difficulty in getting around community due to weakness or other physical limitations. Can perform all self-care activities. Ability to perform role functions limited.

D5 Difficulty in getting around house, can only go out with assistance. Major physical limitations, e.g. can only do light work. Can perform most self-care activities, but needs help getting in and out of the bath. Limited ability to perform role functions.

D6 Confined to a chair, therefore can only get out with assistance. Can only do the lightest of tasks, e.g. switch on the TV. Can feed self, but needs help with all other healthcare activities. Very limited ability to perform role functions.

D7 Confined to bed, needs help with all self-care activities. Minimal ability to perform role functions.

D8 Unconscious.

Discomfort (physical)

P1 No pain.

P2 Slight pain: (a) occasionally, (b) frequently, (c) almost all the time.

P3 Moderate pain: (a) occasionally, (b) frequently, (c) almost all the time.

P4 Severe pain: (a) occasionally, (b) frequently, (c) almost all the time.

P5 Agonising pain: (a) occasionally, (b) frequently, (c) almost all the time.

Distress (emotional)

E1 No distress: very happy and relaxed almost all the time.

E2 Slight distress: happy and relaxed most of the time, but anxious and depressed some of the time.

E3 Moderate distress: anxious and depressed most of the time, but happy and relaxed some of the time.

E4 Severe distress: very anxious and depressed almost all the time.

E5 Extremely depressed: actively suicidal.

To each combination of these states, the following index numbers apply (Table 13).

Table 13

		E1	E2	E3	E4	E5
P1	**D1**	1.000	0.970	0.894	0.791	0.643
	D2	0.990	0.960	0.884	0.781	0.632
	D3	0.971	0.940	0.864	0.762	0.614
	D4	0.946	0.917	0.840	0.738	0.590
	D5	0.917	0.887	0.811	0.710	0.561
	D6	0.885	0.855	0.780	0.678	0.530
	D7	0.838	0.804	0.729	0.628	0.481
P2	**D1**	0.944	0.915	0.838	0.736	0.588
	D2	0.934	0.904	0.828	0.726	0.578
	D3	0.915	0.885	0.810	0.708	0.559
	D4	0.891	0.861	0.785	0.684	0.537
	D5	0.861	0.831	0.756	0.654	0.508
	D6	0.829	0.799	0.724	0.623	0.477
	D7	0.779	0.750	0.675	0.574	0.427
P3	**D1**	0.867	0.837	0.761	0.660	0.513
	D2	0.857	0.827	0.751	0.650	0.503
	D3	0.837	0.808	0.732	0.631	0.485
	D4	0.814	0.784	0.709	0.608	0.461
	D5	0.785	0.755	0.680	0.579	0.433
	D6	0.753	0.723	0.648	0.548	0.402
	D7	0.702	0.674	0.598	0.498	0.353
P4	**D1**	0.714	0.685	0.610	0.510	0.365
	D2	0.703	0.675	0.599	0.499	0.354
	D3	0.685	0.656	0.581	0.481	0.337
	D4	0.661	0.632	0.557	0.458	0.313
	D5	0.632	0.604	0.528	0.429	0.285
	D6	0.601	0.572	0.497	0.399	0.254
	D7	0.551	0.522	0.449	0.350	0.207
P5	**D1**	0.468	0.439	0.365	0.267	0.125
	D2	0.457	0.428	0.355	0.257	0.114
	D3	0.439	0.410	0.337	0.239	0.097
	D4	0.416	0.387	0.314	0.216	0.074
	D5	0.387	0.358	0.285	0.188	0.047
	D6	0.356	0.327	0.255	0.159	0.017
	D7	0.308	0.279	0.207	0.111	−0.030

So, for example, if a patient with chronic rheumatoid arthritis is considered to be in state E4, P3 and D6 their health status is represented by the following descriptions:

E4 Severe distress: very anxious and depressed almost all the time
P3 Moderate pain: (a) occasionally, (b) frequently, (c) almost all the time
D6 Confined to a chair, therefore can only get out with assistance. Can only do the lightest of tasks, e.g. switch on the TV. Can feed self, but needs help with all other healthcare activities. Very limited ability to perform role functions

In reference to Table 13, their health status would be 0.548. This is reading down column E4, going into the P3 area and picking out the number associated with line D6, i.e. 0.548.

Suppose a new care programme enables the patient to move to E1,P1,D3. Then, from Table 13, the patient's new health status is indexed at 0.971. Therefore the patient's quality of life has improved by (0.971 − 0.548) = 0.387 units.

Say the intervention also enables the patient to live an extra seven years. Bringing the estimates of the length of life (seven years) and quality-adjusted life (0.387) together, the patient is estimated to receive 2.709 QALYs.

Imagine another calculation on a paediatric cancer patient reveals that the patient would receive 5.5 QALYs in a new programme, if funded. Can we compare QALYs? If we can, then they can be used to help inform priorities, and resource allocation decisions. *See* **Health; Health index; Index number; QALY.**

Index rebasing
A technique of altering the base date of a set of numbers. Table 14 provides an example using the total cost of NHS prescriptions dispensed by chemists and pharmaceutical contractors between 1970 and 1995.

Table 14 Index rebasing: NHS medicines bill

Year	Total cost	Index with.1970 as base year	Index with 1990 as base year
1970	£209m	100	7
1975	£448m	214	15
1980	£1119m	535	38
1985	£1875m	897	63
1990	£2984m	1428	100
1995	£4711m	2254	158

See **Index number.**

Indifference curve

A locus of points showing all combinations of goods or services that yield the same amount of satisfaction or utility to the consumer. Along the loci the consumer is indifferent to the proportion of which goods or services she has. A standard indifference curve is convex to the origin (Figure 17) but other loci can exist.

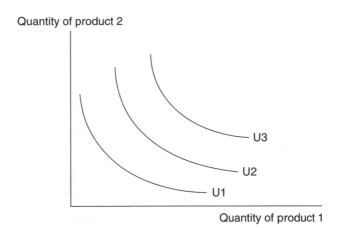

Figure 17 Standard indifference curves

Indifference curves can show the effects of changes in budgets or, with budget loci, the effects of changes in relative prices of the healthcare goods and services for the customer. Generally, a larger budget would allow the customer to reach a higher level of customer satisfaction, i.e. put the customer on a higher indifference curve. Any pattern of preferences can be illustrated by indifference curves.

Figures 17, 18, 19, 20 and 21 show different forms of indifference curves relating to the consumption of two products, 1 and 2. Figure 17 shows the standard indifference curve. The further the curves are from the axis, the greater the utility. Figure 18 shows the utility derived from consuming

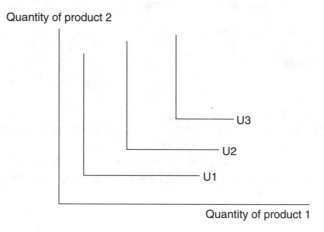

Figure 18 Indifference curves: complementary products

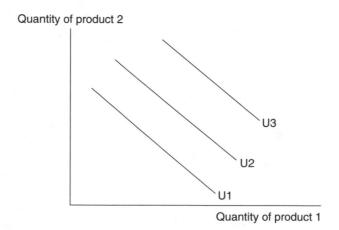

Figure 19 Indifference curves: substitute products

Quantity of product 2

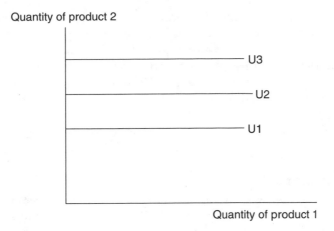

Figure 20 Indifference curves: one product gives no utility

Quantity of product 2

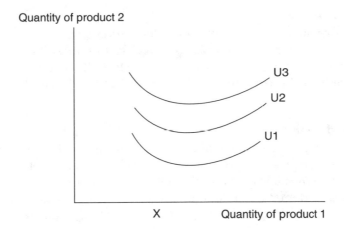

Figure 21 Indifference curves: one product eventually gives no additional utility

products that are perfect complements. An example of this may be a pair of shoes since one of them is generally of little use without the other. We assume that more pairs of shoes brings a person greater utility. Figure 19 shows that two products are perfect substitutes for each other according to the consumer. She would be willing to substitute at a rate of one-to-one between product 1 and product 2. Figure 20 shows that there is one product, product 1, which gives the consumer no utility at all. If the consumer receives no utility from eating red meat, then an example of product 1 will be red meat. In this setting, her only utility is derived from consuming product 2. Figure 21 shows that one of the products, product 1, after point X in the figure, gives the consumer no additional utility.

Difficulties with indifference curves include the following: how to establish their shape; what happens when the individual's indifference curves are discontinuous; can different people's indifference curves be compared; and can different people's indifference curves be added to reflect group or community indifference curves? *See* **Budget locus; Isoquant; Utility.**

Indirect benefit
A benefit such as the patient being able to return to work sooner rather than later as a result of a successful healthcare intervention (e.g. a surgical operation or medication). *See* **Direct benefit; Direct cost; Health measurement pyramid; Indirect cost; Intangible benefit; Intangible cost; Outcome.**

Indirect cost
A cost associated with a healthcare intervention such as patient's time, travel costs or the monetary value of wages lost as a result of sickness or healthcare intervention. *See* **Cost (where costs fall); Direct cost; Human capital method; Indirect benefit; Intangible benefit; Intangible cost.**

Inelastic demand
Occurs when the proportionate change in demand is less than the proportionate change in the price of a healthcare product. Where goods and services have inelastic demand, the seller can hike up the price knowing that although demand may fall, total revenue still rises as demand does not fall very much. *See* **Elasticity; Ramsey pricing principle of public finance.**

Inferior good or service
A type of product whereby as income increases, less of the product is bought. *See* **Income elasticity of demand; Giffen good or service; Merit good or service; Normal good or service; Public good or service.**

Intangible benefit
A benefit associated with a healthcare intervention such as improvements to the patient's social and spiritual life. *See* **Direct benefit; Direct**

cost; Health measurement pyramid; Indirect benefit; Intangible cost; Utility.

Intangible cost

A cost associated with a healthcare intervention such as the patient's pain, anxiety and discomfort. See **Cost (where costs fall); Direct benefit; Direct cost; Human capital method; Indirect benefit; Intangible benefit**.

Interdependent utility function

A mathematical expression which reflects the fact that one person's utility, satisfaction, is dependent on another's. For example, the daughter of a patient undergoing cancer chemotherapy will have her utility affected by the condition of her parent. A husband whose wife is undergoing treatment for multiple sclerosis has his utility affected by her condition. See **Indifference curve; Utility**.

Internal rate of return

That discount rate which makes the present value of income from a project equal to the project's lifetime costs. See **Discount rate; Net present value**.

Internal validity of results

The extent to which the results of a study are valid in that study. See **External validity of results; Systematic review**.

Invisible hand

A term associated with Adam Smith, an 18th-century Scottish polyglot scholar, whereby an unfettered free market would provide the most efficient allocation and distribution of goods and services between willing purchasers and providers. See **Laissez-faire**.

Isoquant

A curve showing all combinations of inputs that yield the same output. See **Isoquant map**.

Isoquant map

A graphical set of isoquants representing different possible outputs from different possible inputs. The highest isoquant (Q3) reflects the maximum output possible from all possible combinations of inputs. Figure 22 shows a set of isoquants using the inputs capital and labour. Isoquants further from the axis represent greater output. Other shapes of isoquants can be set up: their shape depends on the substitution possibilities in production. *See* **Isoquant**.

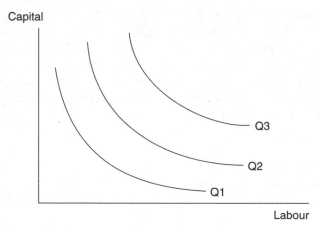

Figure 22 Isoquants

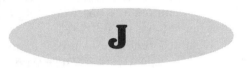

Jarman's index of deprivation

A single number which is said to represent the degree of deprivation of people in a community. The index is made up of eight components:

1 unemployed residents over 16 years of age as a proportion of all economically active residents over 16 years of age in the community;

2 the number of people in households with one or more persons per room as a proportion of all residents in households in the community;

3 the number of households where a pensioner lives alone as a proportion of all households in the community;

4 the number of households where a single parent lives with their offspring alone as a proportion of all households in the community;

5 the number of residents born in the New Commonwealth as a percentage of all residents in the community;

6 the number of children under five years old as a proportion of all residents in the community;

7 the number of persons in households where the economically active head of the household is an unskilled manual worker (socioeconomic group 11) as a proportion of all persons in all households in the community;

8 the number of residents now in the community who had a different residential address outside the community in the previous year as a proportion of all households in the community.

Jarman's index of deprivation is calculated as follows. First, calculate the data for the eight elements (e.g. by census survey). Second, take the square root of each number. Third, use a trigonometric calculation and take what is called the 'arcsine' of the numbers found in the previous step. Fourth, take the Z-scores of the numbers found in step 3. Fifth, apply weights to the resulting data. Component 1 has weight 3.34; component 2 has weight

2.88; component 3 has weight 6.62; component 4 has weight 3.01; component 5 has weight 2.5; component 6 has weight 4.64; component 7 has weight 3.74; and component 8 has weight 2.68.

Sixth, add up the weighted numbers to reveal a single index number, which is the Jarman's index of deprivation. The greater the index number, the greater the deprivation. Whether the components are accurate reflectors of deprivation and whether the method of calculation yields unbiased results is debatable. *See* **Absolute poverty; Carstair's index of deprivation; Department of Employment index for planning; Relative poverty; Townsend's index of deprivation**.

Joint demand

Arises when at least two goods and services are complementary in demand: one is in demand because another related product is in demand. *See* **Joint supply**.

Joint supply

Arises when the creation of one product means the creation of another. *See* **Joint demand**.

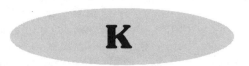

K

Kinked demand curve

An economic model of a market environment. One interpretation of the model is that above a certain market price, if a firm raises its price further, no other supplier will follow; whereas if it lowers its price, other suppliers will follow (Figure 23).

Basically, the market demand curve is kinked at a price, Pk. This could be taken to mean that purchasers are sensitive to price movements above

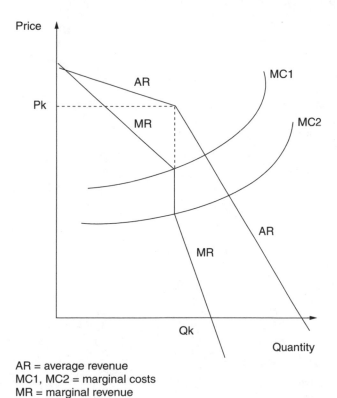

AR = average revenue
MC1, MC2 = marginal costs
MR = marginal revenue

Figure 23 Kinked demand curve

Pk, but less sensitive to price movements below Pk. But the kink may be a result of market regulation. For example, in the UK pharmaceutical price regulation scheme (PPRS), pharmaceutical companies have to receive government permission before they raise prices to the NHS, but do not have to seek permission to lower prices.

At least two interesting economic aspects arise. First, firms facing a kinked demand curve can still maximise profits without needing to know exactly their marginal costs. At best, all they need to know is that their MC curve lies in the range MC1 to MC2. Second, price stability may exist in the market (e.g. around the Pk price).

One unsolved economic issue is how Pk arises in the first place. Maybe an advisory group to the government such as the National Institute of Clinical Excellence could recommend it. Or maybe it reflects the price of the first product in that therapy class. *See* **Average cost; Marginal cost; Marginal revenue; National Institute of Clinical Excellence; Pharmaceutical price regulation scheme; Regulation.**

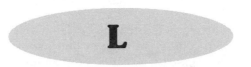

Labour

One of the three factors of production in an economy (the others being land and capital). Labour is both mental and physical activity. *See* **Human capital; Labour force participation rate; Labour theory of value; Labour turnover rate**.

Labour force participation rate

The number of people of working age in employment, divided by the total number of people of working age. For example, if the working age is 18–60 and 40m people are in that age group but only 28m are working, then the labour force participation rate is 70% (28/40). *See* **Labour; Labour theory of value; Labour turnover rate**.

Labour theory of value

The idea that the value of any healthcare product depends on how much labour is embodied in it. The notion stems from the writings of Adam Smith and earlier works of the French physiocrats. It is not, therefore, a Marxist notion although Marxists have fervently championed the idea.

Labour turnover rate

A measure of the number of staff leaving compared to the total number of staff employed in an organisation over a particular period of time. On the one hand, a very high labour turnover rate may represent something inherently wrong with the job(s) as well as inducing extra training and education costs and lowering the opportunities for developing conducive teamwork. On the other hand, a very low labour turnover rate may result in too relaxed a work atmosphere and it can induce complacency.

The labour turnover rate (LTR) is calculated as follows:

$$LTR = \frac{\text{Number of staff leaving in the year}}{\text{Total number of staff employed in the year}}$$

See **Labour; Labour force participation rate; Labour theory of value**.

Laissez-faire

The French term for 'free to act'. The term has been used in economic circles since at least the 18th century to suggest that people and organisations flourish better under a laissez-faire economy than under any other system. This is because freedom to act brings opportunities for personal rewards by individual effort, whereas another system would have regulations by which incentives to act are dampened and regulatory compliance costs incurred. Despite its long history the term still arouses much emotion and debate. It may be more of a philosophical idea than a proven fact. *See* **Invisible hand; Regulation**.

Lakatosian hard-core, protective belt

A Lakatosian hard core is the set of metaphysical beliefs unifying adherents to a research programme. The hard-core beliefs are not testable. Around the hard core there is claimed to exist a 'protective belt' of theories that are testable. *See* **Duhem's irrefutability theory; Falsificationism; Lakatosian research programme; Systematic review**.

Lakatosian research programme

A collection of interconnected theories from a Lakatosian hard core. A progressive Lakatosian research programme captures all facts anticipated by another research programme and provides new facts. A degenerating Lakatosian research programme does not capture all facts anticipated by another research programme or does not provide new facts. *See* **Duhem's irrefutability theory; Falsificationism; Lakatosian hard-core, protective belt; Systematic review**.

Laspeyre index

A method of calculating an index number of a set of numbers. It is based on the initial weights of the factors involved, old and new prices. The calculation for the Laspeyre price index (LPI) is as follows:

$$LPI = \frac{Sum\ P_1 \times W_0}{Sum\ P_0 \times W_0}$$

The Laspeyre price index only needs data on old weights (W_0), old and new prices (P_0 and P_1 respectively). It is used when weights are constant. One way of establishing the weight W_0 is to use initial quantities traded Q_0: set $W_0 = Q_0$. *See* **Fisher's index; Index number; Paasche index**.

Life expectancy

The number of years a person is expected to live. Increases in life expectancy are taken to be a general indicator of improvements in the well-being of people in society. One issue to consider is that improvements in the quality of life should matter as much as changes in life expectancy. Another issue is exactly what contribution healthcare actually makes to life expectancy. *See* **Potential years of life lost**.

Likelihood ratio

A measure comparing the likelihood of a result in one group of patients compared to another. For example, patients may be assigned to a new care regime or usual care; they may or may not be exposed to a risk factor.

Table 15 Likelihood ratio (LR)

	Outcome		
	Event occurs	Event does not occur	Total
New care or exposure	a (1)	b (2)	a + b = (3)
Usual care or not exposed	c (3)	d (4)	c + d = (7)
Totals	a + c = (4)	b + d = (6)	a + b + c + d = (10)

LR+ is the likelihood of an event. Using the symbols in Table 15:

$$LR+ = (a/a + c)/(b/b + d)$$

LR− is the likelihood of no event. Using the symbols in Table 15:

$$LR- = (c/a + c)/(d/b + d)$$

Using the data in Table 15 as an illustration, then, we have:

$$LR+ = (a/a + c)/(b/b + d) = (1/1 + 3)/(2/2 + 4) = (1/4)/(2/6) = 0.75$$

and

$$LR- = (c/a + c)/(d/b + d) = (3/1 + 3)/(4/2 + 4) = (3/4)/(4/6) = 1.25$$

See **Absolute risk; Absolute risk reduction; Incidence; Odds; Odds ratio; Relative risk; Relative risk reduction**.

Likert Scale

A health status measurement scale where patients are asked to express their answer to a question or someone else marks their answer for them. Each degree of agreement is given a numerical value and the total score is the sum of their individual scores.

Suppose the question is 'Do you feel healthy?' One simple set of possible responses is: yes, maybe, no. Another possible set of responses is: yes, mostly, sometimes, not often, no. Many other examples exist (e.g. strongly agree, agree, undecided, disagree, strongly disagree) and the range of possible responses partly depends on the question at hand.

An example of a Likert Scale is the Apgar Score, developed by American anaesthetist Dr Virginia Apgar to determine the general condition of new-born babies. The Apgar Score is based on five criteria (heart rate, respiratory effort, reflex, response to nasal catheter, skin colour) and each criterion can score 0,1 or 2. An example of the scoring is for heart rate: over 100 beats per minute scores 2 points; less than 100 beats per minute scores 1 point; no beat scores 0 points.

Staff in the special care baby unit or the maternity delivery room, or the community midwife if the baby is born at home, usually determine the patient's Apgar Score. An Apgar Score of 8–10 indicates a baby in good condition whereas a score of seven points or less would promote concern for the baby's well-being. *See* **Guttman Scale; Health gain; Health index; Health measurement pyramid; Index of health-related quality of life; QALY; Visual analogue scale**.

Local multiplier

The amount of total expenditure that arises from one tranche of expenditure. For example, when a primary care group decides to purchase £3m more of community services, those services receive this money: in turn they spend some of it and those who receive that spend in turn some of it and so on. The local multiplier can be calculated by first determining the marginal propensities to spend. The first round local multiplier (LM) effect is calculated as follows.

$$LM = \frac{1}{\text{Marginal propensity to spend}}$$

For example, if a primary care group receives £60m in one year and spends £56m, its marginal propensity to spend is (56/60) = 0.933. Therefore the local multiplier is 1/(0.933) = 1.07. For every £1m the primary care group spends, this generates another £0.07m spending in the local economy as a first round effect. *See* **Marginal propensity to consume; Marginal propensity to save.**

Long-run
The time period in which all inputs can be varied. *See* **Short-run.**

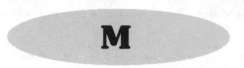

M

Macro economics

A branch of economics that focuses on the economy at large. For example, macro economics can be used to look at the country's expenditure on healthcare. Macro economics is attentive to the total demand and total supply of goods and services. It is concerned with the aggregate rather than the specific individual. *See* **Economics; General equilibrium; Gross domestic product; Gross national product; Micro economics**.

Marginal analysis

A type of economic analysis where the focus of attention is on incremental changes to resources, programmes, cost or outcomes. For example, what is the cost of caring for another Alzheimer's patient? What are the benefits of doing so? Generally, marginal analysis seeks to discover what happens if a little more or a little less of one particular activity takes place. *See* **Externalities; Incremental analysis; Marginal benefit; Marginal cost; Paradox of value; Profit; Programme budgeting; Value for money table; Zero-based budgeting**.

Marginal benefit

The additional benefit that comes from a unit change in output or consumption. More generally, the marginal benefit (MB) is calculated as follows:

$$MB = \frac{\text{Change in total benefit}}{\text{Change in total volume}}$$

See **Marginal cost**.

Marginal cost

The additional cost that comes from a unit change in output or consumption. More generally, the marginal cost (MC) is calculated as follows:

$$MC = \frac{\text{Change in total cost}}{\text{Change in total volume}}$$

See **Cost (type of cost); Marginal benefit.**

Marginal product of capital

The ratio of the change in output divided by the change in capital input by one more unit. *See* **Marginal analysis; Marginal product of labour.**

Marginal product of labour

The ratio of the change in output divided by the change in labour input by one more unit. *See* **Marginal analysis; Marginal product of capital.**

Marginal revenue

The change in revenue that comes from the sale of one more unit. The marginal revenue (MR) calculation is as follows:

$$MR = \frac{\text{Change in total revenue}}{\text{Change in total volume}}$$

See **Marginal analysis; Marginal cost.**

Marginal social benefit

The change in benefit to society that comes from an incremental change in output or consumption. *See* **Analytic perspective; Externalities; Incremental analysis; Marginal social cost; Pigovian subsidy; Social benefit.**

Marginal social cost

The change in cost to society that comes from an incremental change in output or consumption. *See* **Analytic perspective; Externalities; Marginal social benefit; Pigovian tax; Social cost.**

Marginal utility

The change in utility as a result of an incremental change in consumption. *See* **Marginal analysis; Utility**.

Market

A place where healthcare goods and services are traded. The buyers and sellers need not come together physically as they could, for example, trade over the telephone or Internet, by paper or via agents. *See* **Market failure; Market imperfections**.

Market failure

Any departure from optimal market performance. *See* **Market imperfections; Regulation**.

Market imperfections

Factors that make a market different from the economists' model of a perfect market. Examples of imperfections include: externalities, defects or deficits in information, immobility of factors of production, barriers to entry or exit, differentiated products and where suppliers have some degree of control over the price, quality or quantities of the product traded. *See* **Market failure**.

Market power

The influence an organisation or person has over the markets they operate in is a reflection of their market power. Market power, then, is the ability of a person or organisation (e.g. a primary care group) to influence prices, quantities, qualities of healthcare goods and services traded in the market. A monopoly has greatest power (as it is a sole supplier), while firms in a contestable market or a perfectly competitive market have less and no power respectively. Market power may be determined by measures of demand and supply elasticity or, more controversially, by measures of market share and concentration. *See* **Concentration ratio; Contestable market; Market share; Monopoly; Oligopoly; Oligopsony**.

Market share

A measure of how much of a particular market is held by one or more organisations. Market shares can be determined by reference to volume, activity or sales value. *See* **Concentration ratio; Market power**.

Means testing

A method of assessing a person's eligibility for a good, service or payment according to their wealth or income. *See* **Ability to pay; Contributory benefit; Non-contributory benefit.**

Medical Devices Agency

A UK organisation that assesses the safety and performance of medical devices. Unlike medicines, medical devices do not as yet need to receive official licences before they can come on to the market. *See* **Medicines Control Agency; Regulation.**

Medicines Control Agency

A UK organisation that assesses the evidence of the safety, efficacy and quality of medicines prior to a market licensing decision being made. Medicines Control Agency staff critically review the evidence and present their findings to various committees including the Committee on Safety of Medicines (CSM). The CSM then recommends to the UK health ministers (politicians) (the licensing authority) whether and on what terms the product should be licensed on the UK market. Increasingly, however, the European Agency for the Evaluation of Medicinal Products (EMEA) licenses medicines for human consumption in the EU (which includes the UK market). *See* **Barrier to entry; Committee on Safety of Medicines; Medical Devices Agency; Regulation.**

Merit good or service

A merit good or service is one where an organisation, for example a government body, a healthcare team or doctor, believes that the product has greater value in consumption than the actual consumer or others in society think. Less would be consumed if individuals were left to themselves to decide on consuming the product. Education is thought to be a standard example. Vaccinations, e.g. for mumps, measles, rubella, are sometimes considered an example of a merit good or service in healthcare. *See* **Giffen good or service; Inferior good or service; Normal good or service; Public good or service.**

Micro economics

A branch of economics that focuses on the economics of individuals, households, individual enterprise units or individual markets. For example, micro economics can be used on a household's allocation of time and effort in physical exercise. Micro economics can also assess the medicine-prescribing activities and results of specific doctors in a primary care group. Local cancer services may be the subject of a micro economics study. *See* **Economics; Macro economics; Partial equilibrium analysis**.

Minimum efficient scale

The range of output for which costs of production are lowest. Figure 24 shows the minimum efficient production area for endoscopy using the average total cost curve. Alternatively, average variable cost curves can be used to show short-run minimum efficient scales because if a firm does not cover its average variable costs it would soon go out of business. *See* **Average cost pricing; Long-run; Natural monopoly; Short-run**.

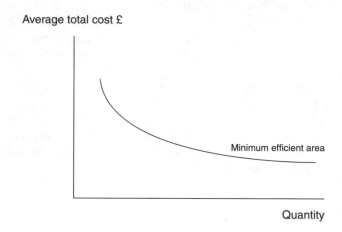

Figure 24 Minimum efficient scale of endoscopy services

Minimum wage

The minimum wage is, for some, an attractive remuneration policy whereby employers cannot pay less than a preset minimum wage. The minimum wage may be written in statute or in an agreement between employers and employees (or their representatives, e.g. unions). Depending on the exact figure, the minimum wage policy can adversely affect employment numbers. In Figure 25, if the minimum wage is set at MW_{high}, then there are more nurses in the market than demand for them. The demand for labour is below the supply and the market is not in equilibrium.

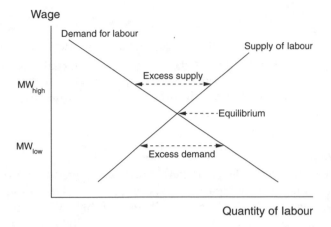

Figure 25 Minimum wage

However if, in Figure 25, the minimum wage is set at MW_{low}, then there are not enough nurses in the market. The demand for labour is above the supply and most companies would pay above the minimum wage to attract and retain nurses. Unions and professional organisations can set out minimum wages policy, as can governments. *See* **Demand curve; Dual labour market hypothesis; Economic rent; Excess demand; Excess supply; Laissez-faire; Partial equilibrium analysis; Regulation; Supply curve.**

Monopolistic competition

An economic description of a market where sellers have control over the prices they charge for their goods and services in the market place. The price differences may arise due to advertising, product differentiation, reputation or supply location. *See* **Monopoly.**

Monopoly

A market situation where there is only one provider of certain goods and services to a market. For example, a primary care group may be served by only one hospital. The monopolist may or may not abuse its monopolistic powers (e.g. extract higher prices, be slow to produce innovations or change or offer lower quality) and it may or may not be inefficient. *See* **Contestable market; Duopoly; Monopsony; Natural monopoly; Oligopoly; Perfect competition.**

Monopsony
A situation where there is only one purchaser of goods and services in a market. The sole purchaser may or may not abuse its monopsonistic powers (e.g. demand lower prices, higher quality, greater volume or push for more innovation). See **Contestable market; Duopsony; Monopoly; Oligopsony; Perfect competition.**

Moral hazard
Arises when the attitudes and behaviour of a person or organisation change once they are covered for the potential costs. For example, once a person becomes insulated from the full costs of their healthcare they may take less care of themselves and consume more healthcare, goods and services than they would otherwise. Once a hospital secures reinsurance for business losses or indemnity against staff malpractice, they may take less care in ensuring business losses or malpractice law suits are minimised. See **Adverse selection; Regulation; User charges.**

Morbidity
A term used to reflect a state of illness. See **Mortality; Quality of life.**

Mortality
A term used to signify death. See **Morbidity.**

Multiple parameter sensitivity analysis
A calculation of how sensitive study results are to changes in more than one parameter or assumption. Suppose a specially organised community nursing service helps avoid inappropriate hospital admissions of elderly patients. Exactly how much the service saves in avoiding inappropriate hospital admissions depends on what would have really happened to the patients in the absence of the service and how much they would have cost if they did go into hospital. Figure 26 shows the amount of hospital expenditure avoided as a result of various combinations of hospital cost and volume. The cost parameter runs from £1 to £2000 per case and the volume parameter from 0% to 100% avoided hospital admissions. If the service avoids X% of the clients going into hospital and the cost would have been p, then the service saves the purchaser no money. If, however, the hospital costs would have been above p, e.g. price q or r, then the purchaser saves £25 000 and £50 000 per year respectively.

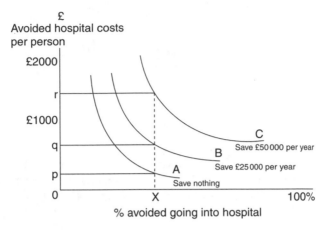

Figure 26 Multiple parameter sensitivity analysis

Curve A shows the combinations of the percentage of patients avoiding hospital and possible hospital costs which yield no savings, on paper, for the purchaser.

Curve B shows the combinations of percentage of patients avoiding hospital and possible hospital costs which yield, on paper, savings of £25 000 per year for the purchaser.

Curve C shows the combinations of percentage of patients avoided going in to hospital and possible hospital costs which, on paper, yield savings of £50 000 per year for the purchaser.

In general, then, areas below curve A reflect situations where the service costs more than hospital entry would, i.e. on paper it makes a loss for the purchaser. Areas above curve A reflect situations where the service costs less than hospital entry would, i.e. on paper it makes a saving for the purchaser. *See* **Sensitivity analysis; Single parameter sensitivity analysis.**

Multiplicative effect

The product of effects from more than one healthcare intervention. Suppose three interventions are provided: T is the kidney transplant, D the kidney transplant anti-rejection medication, E an appropriate patient education video. If T results in t, D in d and E in e and the effects are multiplicative, then the final effect of the three interventions is t × d × e.

One problem here is that two negative results will, when multiplied together, yield a positive result, e.g. 1 × (–2) × (–3) = 6 = 1 × 2 × 3. Another problem is that each effect may have different weights to different people involved in the decision making. *See* **Additive effect.**

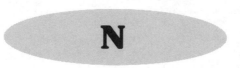

National Framework for Assessing Performance

A new National Health Service (NHS) framework designed to give a clearer and fuller picture of NHS performance. It will cover six areas: health improvement; fair access to services; effective delivery of appropriate healthcare; efficiency; patient and carer experience; and health outcomes of NHS care.

National Health Service trusts

These can currently be defined as public organisations that provide hospital and community healthcare to the UK's NHS. The UK government announced in December 1997 that NHS trusts will:

1 help in the planning of local health services;

2 have a statutory duty to work in partnership with other NHS organisations;

3 help develop new explicit standards for quality and efficiency in local agreements between health authorities, primary care groups and NHS trusts;

4 encourage closer involvement of doctors, nurses and consultants in designing the services and service agreements, with open communication and collaboration, including aligning financial with clinical priorities;

5 develop clinical governance in each NHS trust;

6 share and reinvest efficiency gains to improve services still further;

7 enhance public confidence through openness, improved governance and public commitment to the values and aims of the NHS.

See **Clinical governance; Health authority; National Schedule of Reference Costs; Primary care group.**

National Institute of Clinical Excellence

A new authority in the UK NHS being established to give coherence, authority and prominence to information about clinical and cost-effectiveness of healthcare interventions.

The National Institute of Clinical Excellence (NICE) membership will be drawn from health professionals, the NHS, academics, health economists and patient interests. The Secretary of State for Health, a politician, will appoint a small body of executives and non-executives to the NICE board. The NICE is to be held accountable by the Secretary of State for Health for its resources, delivery of its work programme and for the guidance it produces.

The NICE is a special health authority, which means that it has unique national or supraregional functions which cannot be effectively undertaken by other kinds of NHS bodies. Nevertheless, it is expected to develop relationships at local, regional and national level to help improve the use of resources in the NHS.

It is expected that the NICE will employ a six-step strategy.

Step 1   *Identification and examination:* of medicines, devices and procedures that are likely to have a significant impact on the NHS; examining current practice to identify unjustified variations in use or uncertainty about clinical and cost-effectiveness of healthcare interventions.

Step 2   *Evidence collection:* undertake research to assess the clinical and cost-effectiveness of health interventions.

Step 3   *Appraisal and guidance:* carefully considering the implications for clinical practice of the evidence on clinical and cost-effectiveness and producing guidance for the NHS.

Step 4   *Dissemination:* of the guidance and supporting audit methodologies.

Step 5   *Implementation:* at local level, through clinical governance and other approaches.

Step 6   *Monitoring:* of the impact and keeping advice under review, taking into account the views of patients and their representatives and any relevant new research findings.

In doing this, the NICE will bring together work currently undertaken by other professional organisations in receipt of Department of Health funding. The government has said it will consider developing the role and function of the NICE as it gathers momentum and experience. *See* **Accountability; Analytic perspective; Cost-effectiveness analysis; Due process; Economic assessment decision tree; Governance; Priority setting; Rationing; Regulation; Systematic review; Transparency; Value for money table.**

National Schedule of Reference Costs

Under the current NHS reforms, the government has announced that NHS trusts must publish their costs on a consistent basis and the data will be published in a National Schedule of Reference Costs so that performance on efficiency can be benchmarked. *See* **National Health Service trusts**.

National Service Frameworks

A new set of frameworks for the NHS, setting out what patients can expect to receive from the NHS in major care areas or disease groups. *See* **Accountability; Adaptive expectations; Analytic perspective; Due process; Rational expectations; Regulation; Transparency**.

Natural monopoly

When the optimal size of output from a single firm is as large as the total market demand for the goods or services, then that firm is said to be a natural monopoly. Technical and cost factors therefore preclude the efficient existence of more than one firm in the market place. As the optimal size of the firm is such that the quantity supplied by the firm meets the total market demand for the goods or services, the firm is, in fact, the industry. *See* **Contestable market; Minimum efficient scale; Monopoly; Regulation**.

Need

A healthcare need is a requirement for healthcare. If the need is not identified then it does not become an expressed demand for healthcare. Therefore expressed demand may not capture all healthcare needs. For example, although 10% of the adult male population have erectile dysfunction, only 5% are estimated to present themselves to healthcare professionals. *See* **Demand; Needs assessment; Venn diagram**.

Needs assessment

The calculation of the needs of a person, group of people or organisation. *See* **Demand; Need**.

Net present value

The present value of all future cash flows relevant to a project. Future costs and revenues are brought to today's value by means of a discount rate. The discount factor may be the current interest rate which is considered the opportunity cost of the investment. Sometimes the net present value is called the discounted present value to emphasise the discount element in the calculus. *See* **Discounting; Discount rate; Internal rate of return**.

Non-contributory benefit
Occurs when a benefit is awarded to a person or organisation without the person or organisation necessarily making any contribution to the finance of such. *See* **Contributory benefit; Means testing**.

Non-price competition
Situations where suppliers compete on factors other than price. Examples of non-price competition are: clinical amenity; timeliness (e.g. lower waiting times for treatment); comprehensiveness of medical testing; privacy in hospital; patient briefing and debriefing; better quality or variety of food; recreation facilities such as a reading room available to the patient; pleasant hospital gardens; a clinic room with a pleasant view; ease of access to the hospital; car parking facilities; good communication, rapport and affinity between patient and staff; flexible visiting hours and visiting rules; safety; reliability; reputation; itemised billing; aftersales service; easy access to a dedicated telephone helpline. Non-price competition is important where people perceive that price is not the only or most important factor in the market place. *See* **Price competition**.

Normal good or service
Those for which the demand is indirectly related to the price of the goods or services in question. If the price rises, demand falls and if the price falls, demand rises. *See* **Demand; Elasticity; Giffen good or service; Inferior good or service; Merit good or service; Public good or service**.

Normal profit
The amount of revenue over costs that is just enough to keep the person or organisation in that line of business. *See* **Economic rent; Profit**.

Nottingham Health Profile
The Nottingham Health Profile (Part I) is a collection of questions that seek to establish the physical, emotional and social distress of a person. The questionnaire is self-completed by the patient and is not disease specific. It has six parts relating to: emotional reactions; energy level; physical mobility;

pain; sleep; and social isolation. *See* **EuroQol; Health; Health measurement pyramid; Health profile; Health status; Index of health-related quality of life; QALY; Quality of life; Sickness Impact Profile.**

Null hypothesis
A statement that there is not a specified relationship or difference between factors under study. *See* **Alternative hypothesis; Duhem's irrefutability theory; Falsificationism; Lakatosian research programme; Systematic review.**

Number needed to harm
The number of patients who must be treated in order for one to have an adverse event. For instance, one may have to treat 1000 patients with medication for rheumatoid arthritis before one of them develops related ulcers. *See* **Number needed to treat.**

Number needed to treat
The number of patients who must be treated in order to achieve a result (e.g. avoid one having a clinical event). For example, 30 patients may be needed to treat with one particular medicine to avoid one of them having a myocardial infarction. The number needed to treat (NNT) can be calculated in three ways.

1. NNT is the reciprocal of the absolute risk reduction (ARR): NNT = 1/ ARR. Suppose a primary care group practice nurse is given responsibility for delivering a new myocardial infarction management programme with the purpose of reducing mortality in the group's population. Suppose after one year the ARR = 0.106. Then the NNT is 9.4 (1/0.106). Rounding up to the nearest integer, ten patients have to be treated in the programme to avoid one having a myocardial infarction.

2. The second method depends on knowing the patient expected event rate (sometimes called the control event rate). If we are interested in preventative care then the NNT can be calculated from Table 16 which has eight rows of the control event rate (CER) and nine columns of the odds ratio (OR). It is possible to choose data relevant to local practice to determine the NNT. Suppose, in the prevention of ulcerative colitis, the control event rate is 0.3 and the odds ratio is 0.7. Then reading along row 0.3 and down column 0.7 yields the number 14. Treat 14 patients with the intervention to avoid one having ulcerative colitis.

Table 16 Number needed to treat

OR→ CER ↓	0.5	0.55	0.6	0.65	0.7	0.75	0.8	0.85	0.9
0.05	41	46	52	59	69	83	104	139	209
0.1	21	24	27	31	36	43	54	73	110
0.2	11	13	14	17	20	24	30	40	61
0.3	8	9	10	12	14	18	22	30	46
0.4	7	8	9	10	12	15	19	26	40
0.5	6	7	8	9	11	14	18	25	38
0.7	6	7	9	10	13	16	20	28	44
0.9	12	15	18	22	27	34	46	64	101

3. A third way to calculate the NNT is by reference to Figure 27. Suppose a doctor and geriatrician run a programme to reduce fractured neck of femur. Suppose the programme has a patient expected event rate (PEER) of 2. The PEER reflects the susceptibility of the doctor's patients to the event (in this case, fractured neck of femur). Suppose the preventative intervention has an associated relative risk reduction (RRR) of 10. Plot these points on the PEER and RRR scales respectively, draw a line between the two points and extend the line to the NNT scale. The extended line crosses the NNT scale at 250, suggesting that 250 patients need to be treated in the programme to avoid one fractured neck of femur. If the PEER is 80 and RRR is 3 then, using the same technique as above, 100 patients have to be treated to avoid one patient having a fractured neck of femur. Other combinations of PEERs and RRRs can be used to find other results pertinent to local circumstances.

NNTs can be made more patient specific by converting the NNT to patient-specific NNT (PSNNT). The calculation is that PSNNT = NNT/(f) where f is the patient type factor. On the myocardial infarction programme, if $f = 0.5$ then the PSNNT, using the data above, is 20 (10/0.5).

More generally, if f lies between 0 and 1 then the healthcare professional believes their patient cohort are less susceptible to the event (e.g. myocardial infarction). An f equalling 1 means the healthcare professional believes there are no discernible differences between their patients and the other evidence. If f exceeds 1 this means the health professional believes their patients to be more susceptible to the event (e.g. myocardial infarction).

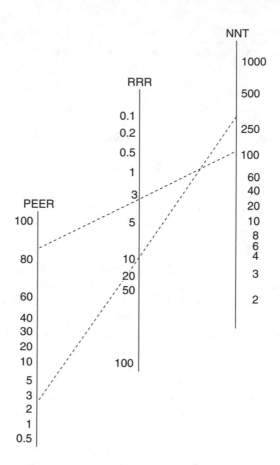

Figure 27 Number needed to treat

Finally, NNTs can be enveloped inside confidence intervals showing, to a degree of certainty (usually 95%), the range of patients needed to treat to achieve a result. Suppose the 95% confidence interval for fractured neck of femur is + or − 40. On these results one would be 95% confident that treating between 210 (250 − 40) and 290 (250 + 40) patients would avoid one having fractured neck of femur. *See* **Absolute risk reduction; Number needed to harm; Odds ratio; Relative risk reduction; Systematic review.**

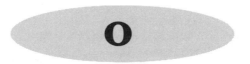

Occupational mobility

Occurs when people trained or skilled in one profession move to another profession. The degree of occupational mobility depends on factors such as the individual's learning abilities, labour market conditions and any overlap in their skills and experiences between the two occupations. For example, some health economists have initially worked in the healthcare sector as nurses, researchers, statisticians, sales executives or managers. Nurses are increasingly involved in prescribing medicines, doctors go into management, some pharmaceutical company sales executives are moving into running disease management programmes. *See* **Barrier to entry; Human capital; Labour turnover rate; Regulation**.

Odds

The ratio of the number of times an event occurs in a group compared to the number of times it does not occur in that group.

Table 17 Odds

	Outcome		
	Event occurs	Event does not occur	Total
New care or exposure	a (1)	b (2)	a + b = (3)
Usual care or not exposed	c (3)	d (4)	c + d = (7)
Totals	a + c = (4)	b + d = (6)	a + b + c + d = (10)

Using the data in Table 17 as an example, then the odds of the event, e.g. stroke, occurring in the new care or exposed group is:

$$ORx = a/b = 1/2 = 0.5$$

and the odds of the event occurring in the usual care or non-exposed group is:

$$ORnotx = c/d = 3/4 = 0.75$$

See **Absolute risk; Absolute risk reduction; Likelihood; Odds ratio; Relative risk; Relative risk reduction.**

Odds ratio

The ratio of two odds. That is, the ratio of the odds that a person in the new care regime or exposed to the risk factor develops the event, e.g. a stroke, compared to the odds that a person in the usual care regime or not exposed to the risk has the event.

Table 18 Odds ratio

	Outcome		
	Event occurs	Event does not occur	Total
New care or exposure	a (1)	b (2)	a + b = (3)
Usual care or not exposed	c (3)	d (4)	c + d = (7)
Totals	a + c = (4)	b + d = (6)	a + b + c + d = (10)

Referring to Table 18, the OR can be written as follows:

$$OR = (a/b)/(c/d)$$

Using the data from Table 18, then:

$$OR = (1/2)/(3/4) = 0.67$$

If the OR = 1 the odds are equivalent. If the OR < 1 the risk of the event is lower in the new care or exposed group than in the other group. If the OR > 1 the risk of the event is higher in the new care or exposed group than in the other group. *See* **Absolute risk; Absolute risk reduction; Likelihood ratio; Odds; Relative risk; Relative risk reduction.**

Off-label use

The prescribing of a medicine for conditions at a dose or for patients that it is not actually officially licensed for. Sometimes called 'beyond the licence'. *See* **Medicines Control Agency.**

Oligopoly

Occurs when a market has only a few suppliers, usually between three and seven. Due to the small number of suppliers, e.g. hospitals in the area, the actions of one supplier can affect and be affected by the actions and reactions of the other suppliers in the market place. *See* **Monopoly; Oligopsony.**

Oligopsony

Occurs when a market has only a few buyers, usually between three and seven. Due to the small number of buyers, e.g. primary care groups in London, Sheffield, North and East Devon, East Riding or in Oxfordshire, the actions of one can affect and be affected by the actions and reactions of other buyers in the market place. *See* **Monopoly; Oligopoly.**

Opportunity cost

The value of the benefits foregone in choosing A rather than B. For example, if the doctor decides to work weekends rather than be with his family then the opportunity cost of working weekends is the value of the benefits that would have come from being with his family. Suppose an NHS hospital decides to use some of its revenue to invest in a new sports and leisure facility for its staff, as recently happened in Oxford. The opportunity cost of this decision is the value of the benefits (e.g. interest) it would have achieved if the next best alternative use for the money was to deposit it in a bank to earn interest. If the government gives £3.5bn more to healthcare than education, the opportunity cost of this decision is the value of the benefits that would have come from the extra spend on education. *See* **Cost (form of cost); Cost (where costs fall).**

Ordinal utility

If utility is ordinal then we can compare one person's utility with another's but not the degree of difference. For example, Mrs Brown receives more utility from taking a medicine once a day than Mrs Walker does from taking another medicine three times a day. Whilst Mrs Brown may indeed receive more utility, we cannot say how much more. *See* **Cardinal utility; Index of health-related quality of life; Normative economics; Positive economics; Priority setting; QALY.**

Outcome

Another term for outputs. For example, improved visual acuity is an outcome from a successful cataract operation. *See* **Health gain; Healthy** years equivalent; Index of health-related quality of life; QALY; Surrogate endpoints.

Over-the-counter medicine

One for which no prescription is required and no pharmacist need be involved in selling or administering the medicine or even on the premises when it is sold. Over-the-counter medicines are available in various retail outlets. *See* **Pharmacy-only medicine; Prescription-only medicine.**

Own price elasticity of demand

A measure of the change in the demand for one product as a result of changes in the price of that product. Suppose nurses receive a 5% wage rise next year. Then the proportionate change in the demand for nurses' services divided by the proportionate change in the price of nurses' services reflects the own price elasticity of demand for nurses' services.

Mathematically, the own price elasticity of demand (OP_{ed}) is calculated as follows:

$$OP_{ed} = \frac{\% \text{ change in demand}}{\% \text{ change in price}}$$

See **Cross price elasticity of demand; Demand; Elasticity; Own price elasticity of supply.**

Own price elasticity of supply

A measure of the change in the supply of one product as a result of changes in the price of that product. For example, the proportionate change in the supply of nurses divided by the proportionate change in the price of their services reflects the own price elasticity for supply of nurses' services. Mathematically, the own price elasticity of supply (OP_{es}) is calculated as follows:

$$OP_{es} = \frac{\% \text{ change in supply}}{\% \text{ change in price}}$$

See **Cross price elasticity of supply; Elasticity; Own price elasticity of demand; Supply.**

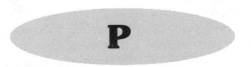

Paasche index

A method of calculating a single number from a set of numbers. It is calculated on the basis of old and new weights (volumes) and old and new prices. The Paasche index (PI) is calculated as follows:

$$PI = \frac{Sum\ P_1 \times W_1}{Sum\ P_0 \times W_0}$$

The Laspeyre price index needs data on old weights (W_0), old and new prices (P_0 and P_1 respectively) whereas the Paasche index needs data on old and new weights (W_0, W_1) and old and new prices (P_0, P_1). Weights can be established by using quantities traded: $W_0 = Q_0$, $W_1 = Q_1$. *See* **Fisher's index; Index number; Laspeyre index.**

PACT

First established in 1988, Prescription Analysis and CosT (PACT) is a system of providing information (based on prescriptions dispensed in the NHS) on what a general practitioner (GP), working in England or Wales, has prescribed in a period (e.g. the last three months). PACT provides information on the GP's practice and shows how they compare with more aggregated information (e.g. at primary care group, health authority or national level). PACT standard reports are automatically sent to every GP to whom the data refer. More detailed information is sent to GPs on request. PACT information is also provided to health authority medical advisers and has been used in prescribing analysis.

A standard report includes: information on practice prescribing costs; how these compare to health authority and national costs; the number of items the practice prescribes; prescribing data by therapeutic group (e.g. gastrointestinal, cardiovascular, respiratory, central nervous system, endocrine, musculoskeletal and joint disorders); own dispensing (if the doctor is allowed to prescribe and dispense medicines, e.g. in a GP practice in a rural area); the practice's profile (e.g. patient list size, number of patients over 65 years of age); prescribing attributed to the GP's trainees or deputies. PACT allows GPs to view and review their prescribing practice; monitor the influence of practice policies (e.g. their use of restricted lists); and compare their performance with others. One main disadvantage of PACT is that it does not provide any diagnosis information; therefore we do not know exactly what the medicine was prescribed for. *See* **ASTRO-PU; DDD; General Practice Research Database; STAR-PU**.

Paradox of value
Exists where some goods and services essential to life have a lower market value than other goods and services which are not deemed essential to life. For example, water is essential to life but has a low market value, whereas diamonds are not essential to life but have a high market value. *See* **Marginal analysis**.

Paradox of voting
The situation whereby in a system of majority voting, individual preferences cannot be fully reflected in community preferences. If Mrs Green votes for A,B,C, Mr Brown for B,C,A and Ms Red for C,A,B then any majority voting system cannot reflect all individuals' preferences. Sometimes called Arrow's impossibility theorem. *See* **Priority setting; Transitivity**.

Pareto efficiency
A situation is said to be Pareto efficient if it is not possible to make someone better off without making someone else worse off. In a Pareto-efficient situation two types of efficiencies occur: technical efficiency (inputs are being used in the most efficient way) and allocative efficiency (outputs provide the highest possible utility). Sometimes called Pareto optimal. *See* **Pareto improvement; Pareto optimal**.

Pareto improvement
Occurs when someone is made better off and no one is made worse off. *See* **Equilibrium; Pareto efficiency; Pareto optimal**.

Pareto optimal
Occurs when it is not possible to make someone better off without making someone else worse off by a reallocation of incentives or resources. Sometimes called Pareto efficiency. *See* **Pareto efficiency**.

Partial equilibrium analysis

Occurs when individual markets, but not all markets, are assessed for their state of equilibrium. For example, an analysis of the cystic fibrosis market represents a partial equilibrium analysis. *See* **Equilibrium; General equilibrium; Micro economics.**

Per capita

A term used to denote calculations based on population numbers. For example, if a primary care group's expenditure is £60m per annum and there are 100 000 people covered in the group, then healthcare expenditure is £600 per capita. Not everyone in the 100 000 will have used healthcare goods and services while those who have received healthcare may have received different care packages, generated different actual care costs and received different health gains.

More generally, in 1986 healthcare expenditure per capita in the UK was £390 and in 1996 it was £830 in cash terms. Even allowing for inflation, the change in per capita expenditure does not mean that all individuals in the UK are better off in terms of health status in 1996 as compared to 1986.

Perfect competition

An economic concept of a market with the following attributes: all firms are price takers; no firm can affect the market price; a homogeneous product or service is offered; people have perfect information about market conditions; there are no barriers of entry to or exit from the market; and there is free movement of all factors of production. *See* **Barrier to entry; Barrier to exit; Imperfect competition; Imperfect oligopoly; Monopoly; Oligopoly; Perfect oligopoly.**

Perfect oligopoly

An economic concept of a market where there are a small number of firms in the market (say seven) each producing indistinguishable goods or services but possibly selling them at different prices. The only dimension on which they can compete, therefore, is price. *See* **Imperfect oligopoly; Monopoly; Perfect competition; Price competition.**

Pharmaceutical price regulation scheme

The UK pharmaceutical price regulation scheme (PPRS) is an agreement between the Department of Health and the Association of the British

Pharmaceutical Industry (ABPI) conditioning the incentives and rewards in sales of medicines to the UK NHS. It is currently a voluntary agreement and applies to any company supplying medicines to the NHS whether or not they are members of the ABPI. New medicines, those with a new product licence from the Medicines Control Agency, are exempt from the price control element of the scheme for the first five years of their UK market life. Generic medicines, medicines on private prescriptions and non-prescription medicines are also exempt.

The stated objectives of the 1993–98 pharmaceutical price regulation scheme (running from October 1993 to September 1998) are:

1 to secure the provision of safe and effective medicines for the NHS at reasonable prices;

2 to promote a strong and profitable pharmaceutical industry in the United Kingdom capable of such sustained research and development expenditure as should lead to the future availability of new and improved medicines;

3 to encourage in the United Kingdom the efficient and competitive development and supply of medicines to pharmaceutical markets in this and other countries.

The PPRS has four parts. One part regulates the rate of return on capital employed that pharmaceutical companies can keep on their sales to the NHS (the 1993–98 agreed band was 17–21%). A second part conditions price rises of medicines. A third part regulates the amount of pharmaceutical advertising expenditure that can be considered as a cost of supplying medicines to the NHS (9% of sales in the 1993–98 agreement). The fourth part conditions the amount of R & D expenditure that can be attributed to costs of medicines sold to the NHS (20% of sales in the 1993–98 agreement). While there is no robust evidence that the scheme is or is not a success, it is only one of the regulatory instruments used to condition the pharmaceutical market. *See* **Efficiency; Kinked demand curve; Price cap regulation; Reduced form regulation; Reference pricing; Regulation; Yardstick pricing.**

Pharmacy-only medicine

One for which no prescription is required, but a pharmacist must either deliver the medicine to the patient (or their agent) or be in the pharmacy when the medicine is given to the patient or their agent (e.g. the patient's spouse). Pharmacy-only medicines are those which the licensing authorities believe are safe enough to be purchased without the advice or oversight of a doctor, dentist or nurse but which require some professional supervision (by the pharmacist). *See* **Medicines Control Agency; Over-the-counter medicine; Prescription-only medicine.**

Pigovian subsidy
A fiscal intervention, e.g. a tax allowance, to help promote the production and use of a particular product when the product in question has external benefits; for example, tax credits on private pensions. *See* **Efficiency; Externalities; Merit good or service; Pigovian tax; Social benefit; Social cost.**

Pigovian tax
A fiscal intervention to help lower the production and use of a particular product, when the product in question has external costs. *See* **Efficiency; Externalities; Pigovian subsidy; Social benefit; Social cost.**

Placebo
A medicine which is indistinguishable from another in terms of packaging, taste, smell, texture, form, colour and size. The only difference between the two products is that the placebo medicine does not have the active pharmacological ingredients in it. *See* **Hawthorne effect; Hello-goodbye effect; Placebo effect.**

Placebo effect
Suppose a new medicine is to be tested for its safety, efficacy and efficiency. Patients may be randomly allocated to one of two groups: group 1 who receive the medicine and group 2 who receive the placebo. Measured results from group 2's consumption of the placebo are called placebo effects. *See* **Hawthorne effect; Placebo.**

Play the winner rule
A principle that the next patient receives healthcare intervention depending on the results of the intervention for the current patient. If the results from the intervention in the current patient are positive then the next patient receives the same intervention; if the results are negative then the next patient receives the alternative treatment.

Positive list

A list of goods and services which can be used by an organisation or individual. Most hospital pharmacies have a list of medicines that can be used in the hospital. Health insurers may have positive lists of medicines that they will pay for in their schemes. The UK government has a list of medicines that cannot be provided or paid for under the NHS. It also has a list of medicines that can be used, i.e. a positive list (Department of Health's monthly publication *The Drug Tariff*).

It can be suggested that positive lists encroach upon clinical freedom and therefore abrogate the health professional's ability to give the patient the best care. The nature of the list, the goods and services on the list, entry to the list and exit from the list are important issues for healthcare.

There is no robust reason why organisations need have exactly the same substantive and procedural positive lists. For example, across the UK, NHS trust hospitals have different lists of medicines they will pay for. Primary care groups can also be expected to develop their own positive lists.

Positive lists have generally been applied to pharmaceuticals but they also apply to medical technology and diagnostic equipment. More recently, there is a trend towards developing positive lists of procedures, medical and surgical. *See* **Blacklist; Formulary; Negative list**.

Potential Pareto improvement

Said to exist when a particular change would leave at least one person better off without making anyone else worse off in the economy. *See* **Compensating principle; Pareto efficiency; Pareto improvement**.

Potential years of life lost

An estimate of the number of years of life lost as a result of premature death. *See* **Life expectancy; Years of life lost**.

Poverty trap

A situation whereby doing more work leads to one being worse off. The existence of a poverty trap can relate to the welfare and transfer payments someone receives but would have to relinquish if they engaged in more work. It is closely related to the unemployment trap but there are subtle differences, one being that the poverty trap can exist even if one is employed.

The effects of the poverty trap on health and the economy are complex and multifaceted. If there is a causal relationship between poverty and ill health, then people in the poverty trap and their dependants may have a greater susceptibility to ill health than others. They are therefore less likely to be able to escape from the trap and more likely to need healthcare. *See* **Healthy worker effect; Unemployment trap.**

Power of a test
The probability that a null hypothesis will be rejected if it is in fact false. *See* **Null hypothesis; Type II error.**

Prescription-only medicine
One for which the patient requires a prescription from an authoritative source, e.g. a doctor, dentist or nurse, before they can receive the medicine, e.g. from a dispensing pharmacist. *See* **Over-the-counter medicine; Pharmacy-only medicine.**

Present value
The value today of future revenue. *See* **Discounting; Discount rate; Internal rate of return; Net present value.**

Prevalence rate
The prevalence rate (PR) is the number of cases of a disease present, divided by the number of people exposed to the risk of developing the disease during that time period:

$$PR = \frac{\text{Number of cases}}{\text{Population exposed}} \times 1000$$

See **Incidence rate.**

Price cap regulation
A regulatory system whereby prices are allowed to rise by up to a certain amount, the level of the cap, over a particular period of time.

Price cap regulation has become a common instrument in regulating the UK utility industries (e.g. gas, electricity, water) where it is known as the 'RPI-X'. Under RPI-X certain prices are allowed to rise by an amount RPI less a factor X. RPI is the retail price index and X is a deflating factor.

Various points have to be noted with price cap regulation. First, how are initial prices set? A high initial price, with respect to costs, makes it easier to keep within the price cap. What prices are to be capped? Wholesale, retail? What goods and services are to be capped? How long does the cap last? What factors will lead to a change in the cap? Suppose profits rose substantially, would that signal efficiency or inefficiency? Would rising or falling profits lead to a change in the price cap? If so, this can obviate the incentives and credibility of the regulation. How is X determined? Is the RPI the most suitable index to use? *See* **Rate of return regulation; Reduced form regulation; Reference pricing; Regulation.**

Price competition

Occurs when alternative suppliers vie for custom on the basis of the price of the healthcare product they are supplying. *See* **Non-price competition; Perfect competition.**

Price–consumption curve

A locus of points that show how consumption changes when the product's price changes, holding other factors, e.g. income, constant. It can be determined by the use of indifference curves and budget loci. Figure 28 gives an example.

If the price of product A falls, then the budget lines move out from BL1 to BL2 or BL3 and utility rises from U1 to U2 or U3 respectively. The price–consumption curve is the locus of points where the utility curves U1, U2,

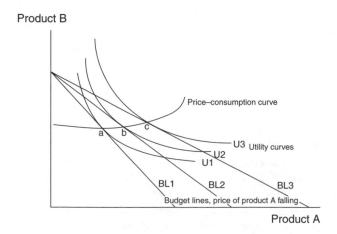

Figure 28 Price–consumption curve

U3 are tangential to the budget lines BL1, BL2, BL3 respectively, e.g. points a, b, c. *See* **Budget locus;** *Ceteris paribus;* **Income–consumption curve; Income effect; Indifference curves; Slutsky decomposition; Substitution effect; Utility.**

Price discrimination

Occurs when a supplier charges a different price to different customers for the same healthcare product. The customers may differ according to their price sensitivity, the volume of their purchases, geographic location or a time factor. For example, a NHS hospital trust may charge private health insurers different rates than a local primary care group. *See* **Elasticity; Product differentiation.**

Price elasticity of demand

A measure of the responsiveness of demand to changes in the price of the product. A high price elasticity of demand shows that purchasers are price sensitive, whereas a low price elasticity of demand shows purchasers are less sensitive to price. *See* **Cross price elasticity of demand; Cross price elasticity of supply; Demand curve; Elasticity; Kinked demand curve; Own price elasticity of demand; Own price elasticity of supply; Price elasticity of supply.**

Price elasticity of supply

A measure of the responsiveness of supply to changes in the price of the product. A high price elasticity of supply shows that producers are price sensitive, whereas a low price elasticity of supply shows that producers are less price sensitive. *See* **Cross price elasticity of demand; Cross price elasticity of supply; Elasticity; Own price elasticity of demand; Own price elasticity of supply; Price elasticity of demand; Supply curve.**

Primary care

Family health services provided by family doctors, dentists, pharmacists, community nurses, midwives, health visitors, optometrists and ophthalmic medical practitioners. *See* **Primary care group.**

Primary care group

New organisations in the NHS which will bring together primary care professionals (e.g. family doctors and community nurses).

Primary care groups are expected to include around 50 family doctors in general practice, cover an average of 100 000 people in their area and receive around £60m per annum. Their funding will be in the form of unified primary care group budgets (cash-limited funds), used to cover hospital and community health services, prescribing and infrastructure (e.g. a proportion of the cost of their practice staff, premises and computers). This is the first time in the history of the NHS that doctors in primary care will have to conduct their NHS business within cash-limited funds.

According to UK government documents, the functions of the primary care groups are to:

1 *contribute* to the health authority's health improvement programme on health and healthcare, helping to ensure that this reflects the perspective of the local community and the experience of patients;

2 *promote* the health of the local population, working in partnership with other agencies;

3 *commission* health services for their populations from the relevant NHS trusts, within the framework of the health improvement programme;

4 *monitor* performance against the service agreements they have with the NHS trust;

5 *develop* primary care by joint working across practices, sharing skills, providing a forum for professional development, audit and peer review, assuring quality and developing the new approach to clinical governance and influencing the deployment of resources, for general practice locally;

6 better *integrate* primary and community healthcare services;

7 *work more closely* with Social Services.

Primary care groups came into existence in 1999 and will develop over time, learning from existing arrangements, their own and others' experience. There are four basic types of primary care group:

Type 1 As a minimum, *support the health authority* in commissioning care for its population, acting in an advisory capacity.

Type 2 *Take devolved responsibility* for managing the budget for healthcare in their area, formally as part of the health authority.

Type 3 Become established as *free-standing bodies* accountable to the health authority for commissioning care.

Type 4 Become established as *free-standing bodies* accountable to the health authority for commissioning care and *with added responsibility* for the provision of community health services for their population.

It is expected that most primary care groups will move in to type 3 or 4 over time. *See* **Accountability; Clinical governance; Due process; Health authority; Health action zones; Health improvement programme; Marginal analysis; National Health Service trusts; National Service Frameworks; Primary care; Programme budgeting; Transparency; Virement**.

Principal–agent problem

Occurs when it is impossible to write up contracts between principals and agents (e.g. patients and primary care group doctors) specifying every possible eventuality whereby the agent will act in the principal's best interest.

Priority setting

The business of establishing a ranking of preferences by seniority. Priorities can be calculated in different ways: examples include protocols, weights, mathematical formulae or voting.

Priority protocols The following example comes from City and Hackney Health Authority in London. A set of criteria or protocols can be used to help explicitly establish the ranking of preferences. Each possible purchase can be assessed according to a seven-point protocol and for each point, there is a possible range of scoring (xx–yy):

1 Robustness/implementability of proposal (0–3)

2 Promotion of equity (0–1)

3 Evidence of effectiveness/cost-effectiveness (0–2)

4 Collaboration with/integration with primary care (0–3)

5 Prioritised by Community Health Council (0–1)

6 Prioritised by General Practitioner (GP) or GP forum (0–1)

7 Other possible/more appropriate sources of funding (–5–0)

For criterion 1, the more robust or implementable the proposal, the higher is its number in the range between 0 and 3. For criterion 3, if the evidence is strong that the intervention will be cost-effective, the higher is its number in the range between 0 and 2. For criterion 7, if alternative sources of funding can be found the lower the priority, or the lower the reason, for City and Hackney to pay for it.

Priority weights The following example comes from Wandsworth Health Authority in London. Each possible purchase can be assessed according to five questions and each question has a weight attached (zz):

1 Potential for health gain (40)

2 Improves quality of service (20)

3 In accordance with local views (20)

4 Achievability in current year (15)

5 In accordance with national and regional priorities (5).

The exercise is to establish the data for each question and use the weights to calculate the priority figure. Notice that the weight for the potential for health gain is eight times greater than the weight for whether or not the healthcare intervention is in accordance with regional or national priorities.

Priority formulae The following example comes from Gwynedd Health Authority in Wales. Each possible purchase can be assessed according to scores from four questions:

1 Number of people benefiting from the healthcare intervention

2 The benefit per person

3 The quality of evidence available or yet to be collected

4 The degree of difficulty (e.g. Health Commissioner time, cost).

The calculation is as follows:

$$\text{Priority rating} = \frac{A \times B \times C}{D}$$

Gwynedd Health Authority argued that 'No system (of priority setting) should pretend that it represents the ultimate truth'. The authority also argued that a system of priority setting, however imperfect, would help show how little is known of what is currently bought. *See* **Accountability; Due process; Paradox of voting; Rationing; Systematic review; Transparency.**

Prisoners' dilemma

A situation whereby welfare is maximised if people have as much concern for each other as they do for themselves.

Process utility

The level of satisfaction that a person receives from going through the process of a healthcare intervention. Process utility differs from outcome utility which is the satisfaction received from the outcomes of healthcare intervention. For example, a kidney transplant patient or a breast cancer patient can be expected to receive degrees of satisfaction from the procedures and steps that are followed in their care. The process utility may or may not be positive, i.e. if negative, this signals the patient's dissatisfaction with the process of care received. *See* **Externalities; Indifference curve; National Service Frameworks; Outcome; QALY; Utility.**

Producer's surplus

The extra revenue a producer receives over and above the minimum that the producer would be willing to take for providing a particular healthcare product. For example, at £300 each, the producer would be willing to supply three units. At £200 each, the producer is willing to supply two units; at £100 each, the producer is willing to supply one unit. If the producer can sell at £300, they will sell three units. This is despite the fact that they were willing to sell one unit at £100 and two units at £200. More generally, in Figure 29 the producer's surplus is represented by triangle ABC. The

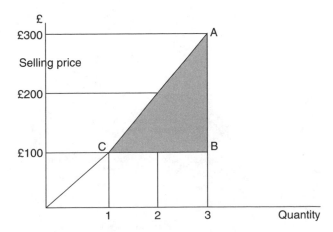

Figure 29 Producer's surplus

monetary value of the producer's surplus is, in this example, of the value of £200 (the area of the triangle ABC). *See* **Consumer's surplus; Economic rent**.

Product differentiation

The practice of making one's product distinctive from another's. The distinctions may be real or psychological. The differences may be technical, physical, clinical or in terms of price, place or speed of access to the service. Examples include: slow-release medicines compared to once-a-day medicines; skin patches compared to tablets; differences in strengths or pack size of the product. Products can also be differentiated by trade marks, brand names and advertising or by building a reputation associated with the product. A fully differentiated healthcare product is one for which the purchaser or consumer believes that there is no practical or satisfactory substitute available. *See* **Cross price elasticity of demand; Elasticity of substitution; Substitutes**.

Product lifecycle

The notion that all heathcare goods and services follow a cycle in life starting with product conception, product birth, growth, maturity and then demise of the product. Medicines follow product lifecycles. The length of the product lifecycle depends on the demand for the product, its therapeutic and technical gains over substitute products, the time it takes for alternatives to come to the market, tastes and fashion. Figure 30 gives an illustration.

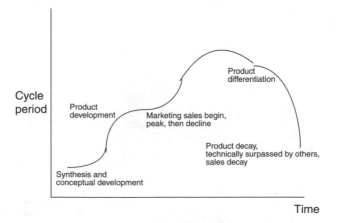

Figure 30 Product lifecycle

Production function

A mathematical formula expressing the relationship between inputs, processes and outputs. *See* **Production possibility curve**.

Production possibility curve

A locus of combinations of inputs that yield the same output. Figure 31 gives an example of a production possibility curve of two healthcare services. See production possibility frontier for further illustrations and discussion. *See* **Production function; Production possibility frontier**.

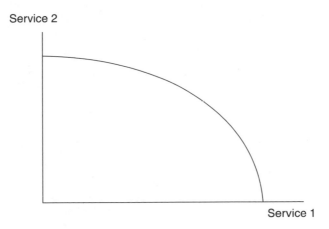

Figure 31 Production possibility curve

Production possibility frontier

The locus of inputs that yield maximum possible output that the health-care system can produce with a given set of resources. The resources are categorised as land, labour and capital. Figure 32 shows the production possibility frontier of an NHS hospital trust. Suppose there is interest in hernia operations compared to all other goods and services the hospital can provide. If the hospital produces X hernia operations and Y other goods and services then it is working below its production possibility frontier. In Figure 32 it would be at a point such as 1. This means that the hospital is not working as efficiently or effectively as it could with its set of resources.

Suppose as a result of the recent NHS reforms, a hospital's management and the rest of the staff decide to change some of their working practices in order to provide X^2 hernia operations but still only Y other goods and services. Then it has moved onto its production possibility frontier; in Figure 32, the hospital would be at point 2. The hospital could have changed to provide X hernia operations and Y^3 other goods and services. Then, it would have moved to point 3. Either way, it would move to its production possibility frontier.

Given the set of resources, the hospital cannot go beyond its production possibility frontier. That is, it cannot reach a point such as 4 in Figure 32. At best, it can produce on its frontier. It can also produce at points under its frontier.

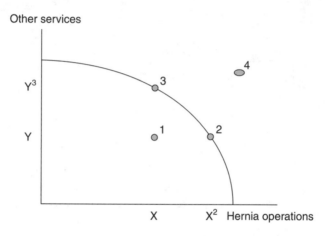

Figure 32 Production possibility frontier (1)

In Figure 32, the slope of the frontier or curve can be used to illustrate the trade-off between hernia operations and all other goods and services. The greater the slope, the greater the trade-off.

A production possibility frontier can be changed if the hospital's set of resources changes. For example, more staff in all services may enable the production possibility frontier to move from PPF^1 to PPF^2, as in Figure 33. On the new production possibility frontier, the hospital can now produce X^4 hernia operations and Y^4 other services, as indicated by point 4 in Figure 33.

More staff in only one speciality, e.g. hernia support staff, may be able to move the production possibility frontier out from PPF^1 to PPF^3, as seen in

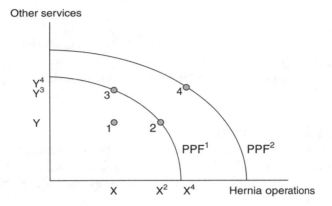

Figure 33 Production possibility frontier (2)

Figure 34. The hospital can, for example, produce X^5 hernia operations and Y^5 other services, e.g. at point 5 on the new production possibility frontier PPF^3 indicated in Figure 34.

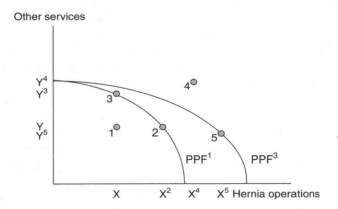

Figure 34 Production possibility frontier (3)

The production possibility frontier is sometimes called the production possibility curve. *See* **Production possibility curve; Stochastic frontier analysis**.

Profit
The excess amount of revenue over and above costs. It has also been defined as the amount necessary to keep an entrepreneur in a particular activity. See **Economic rent; Normal profit; Profit-maximising principle**.

Profit-maximising principle
Profits are maximised when marginal cost equals marginal revenue. It therefore depends on identifying, measuring and matching the marginal costs and revenue. See **Economic rent; Marginal cost; Marginal revenue; Normal profit; Profit**.

Programme budgeting
A technique that determines the programme of healthcare goods and services being bought or sold. For example, a primary care group can use programme budgeting to show the distribution of their expenditure on healthcare goods and services, to organisations, by groups of patients (e.g. age, sex profiles), by staff mix or to illustrate their debt/creditor detail.

Programme budgeting can be used with marginal analysis to help decide how to improve the use of scarce resources.

The technique is neither new nor unique to healthcare. Programme budgeting and marginal analysis were used in the 1960s in defence, space exploration and law and order in the US but abandoned in the early 1970s. They were also used in local government authorities in the UK, e.g. in Coventry, but the exercise was generally discarded in the mid-1970s. See *British Medical Journal* **guidelines for economic evaluation; Compliance cost assessment; Cost–benefit analysis; Cost-effectiveness analysis; Cost-minimisation analysis; Cost–utility analysis; Economic assessment decision tree; Guidance on Good Practice in the Conduct of Economic Evaluations of Medicines; Marginal analysis; Value for money table; Zero-based budgeting**.

Progressive tax
Exists when the tax paid as a proportion of, say, income is higher the more one earns. See **Proportional tax; Regressive tax**.

Proportional tax

Exists when the tax paid as a proportion of, say, income is the same regardless of the amount of income earned. *See* **Progressive tax; Regressive tax**.

Public good or service

A product which has certain associated characteristics that distinguish it from other goods or services. The essential characteristics of public goods are as follows:

1 If the product is provided to one person, no one else can be excluded from it (non-excludability).

2 One persons' consumption of the product does not preclude nor diminish any other person's consumption of it (non-rivalry).

Standard examples of public goods have included the service of a lighthouse to seafarers, the provision of military defence of a country, the provision of law and order in a community, the provision of street lighting.

It is usually thought that the public purse (government) should pay for the provision of public goods or services since no individual has any incentive to pay for them. Yet it is debatable whether, strictly, any public goods or services do actually exist and it is not necessarily true that the public purse should pay for such. *See* **Giffen good or service; Inferior good or service; Merit good or service; Normal good or service; Ramsey pricing principle of public finance**.

Purchasing power parity

The notion that the equilibrium exchange rate between trading countries will equate with the purchasing power of people and organisations in the trading countries. For example, if the equilibrium exchange rate between the UK and US is £1 = $1.60, under purchasing power parity, £1 spent in the UK can buy essentially the same healthcare goods and services as $1.60 would in the US. *See* **Terms of trade**.

QALY

A quality-adjusted life-year (QALY) is a measure of health outcome, a combination of the change in quality of life and the change in life expectancy caused by some healthcare intervention. Suppose a new medicine allows a patient to live five more years but only in a state of health that is considered half as good as perfect health. Then the QALY is 2.5 (5 × 0.5).

Suppose the healthcare intervention raises the patient's quality of life and extends their length of life by five years. Then using a hypothetical example, Figure 35 shows the length of life and quality of life for a person who does not have the healthcare treatment (curve X) compared to their possible scenario if they did have the healthcare intervention (curve Y). The total area between curves X and Y represents the total QALY. This diagram shows that the healthcare intervention yields a positive total QALY.

A high QALY can suggest that the person has more to gain from the intervention than someone with a lower QALY. If QALYs are comparable then they may be used to help inform resource allocation in healthcare, e.g. in priority setting.

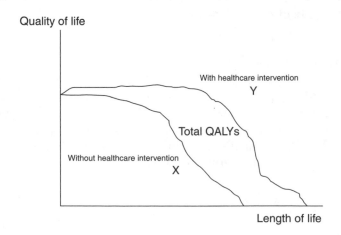

Figure 35 QALY

As QALYs are determined as the product of quality of life and length of life there is a pertinent question about how to measure quality of life. It has to be pointed out that the QALY could be derived from various different quality of life measures and therefore we could have different QALYs for exactly the same person undergoing the exactly the same healthcare intervention.

The index of health-related quality of life has been used but so too have other indices, including the Kaplan index of well-being in the US. Due to the profusion of measures of quality of life, it is difficult to identify a figure that can represent quality of life and so be used in the calculation of a QALY. *See* **Health measurement pyramid; Healthy years equivalent; Index of health-related quality of life; Outcome; Quality-adjusted survival time; Quality-adjusted time without symptoms or toxicity; Quality of life**.

Quality-adjusted survival time

Quality-adjusted survival time (QAST) is a measure of the change in quality of life multiplied by the change in life duration. For example, orlistat, an anti-obesity medication, in combination with a hypocaloric diet including 30% of calories in fat and multivitamin supplements, may enable an obese patient to live five more years than they would otherwise and at a lower weight (with concomitant improvements in their quality of life). To get the QAST, we would need to identify and measure the change in quality of life and then multiply it by the survival time of the patient. *See* **Healthy years equivalent; QALY; Quality-adjusted time without symptoms or toxicity; Quality of life**.

Quality-adjusted time without symptoms or toxicity

Quality-adjusted time without symptoms or toxicity (Q-TWiST) is a measure of the quality of a person's life during which period they are free from symptoms or toxicity. For example, Q-TWiSTs have been used in patients treated for breast cancer. *See* **QALY; Quality-adjusted survival time; Quality of life**.

Quality of life

There is no universal definition of what quality of life is, what factors determine it or how to measure it accurately. Quality of life is an important driver of the demand for healthcare. It is contingent on one's own condition but it can also be affected by the perceptions of others' conditions. Thus it is a mixture of absolute and relative factors.

Some of the factors determining quality of life include: employment, the environment, family welfare, healthcare, education, sanitation, housing, income, perceptions, prospects, public health, recreation, feelings of safety, security, spiritual beliefs and practices, food consumption, transport. It is therefore obvious that healthcare may only have a limited role in changing or maintaining one's quality of life.

One definition of quality of life is:

an individual's perception of their position in life in the context of the culture and value systems in which they live and in relation to their goals, expectations, standards and concerns. It is a broad ranging concept affected in a complex way by the person's physical health, psychological state, level of independence, social relationships, and their relationships to salient features of their environment.

Another definition of quality of life is in relation to the degree to which a person accomplishes life goals. A third definition of quality of life relates it to one's endowment and the effort made on one's behalf by family and society.

Many attempts continue to be made to establish the impact of healthcare on quality of life. These measurement instruments are a reduced form of measuring quality of life. Reduced-form measurement is useful if the excluded factors either play an unimportant role or are insignificant in the person's quality of life. The reduced-form measures can, at best, be seen as important parts of the wider picture.

If the measure of quality of life has more than one component, then are all the components of the same weight or of equal value? The answer to this will depend on to whom the factors are important. For example, the patient may not think that climbing stairs is as important as being able to wash, dress or feed oneself.

Quality of life measures help generate information on which resource allocation decisions can be made. For example, if course A yields a higher quality of life than course B, then healthcare priorities can be based on such. However, priorities should also take into account the costs of courses A and B in addition to any claimed and measured benefits. *See* **Analytic perspective; Health; Health gain; Health index; Health measurement pyramid; Health profile; Health status; Index of health-related quality of life; Outcome; QALY; Quality of life index.**

Quality of life index

The quality of life index (QoLi) is a set of questions that aim to identify and measure the general quality of life of a person and summarise that in a single number. The questions relate to factors over the previous week. There are five categories of life in the questionnaire: activity, daily living, health, support and outlook. To each question the answer has to be 0, 1 or 2, with 2 reflecting the best quality of life and 0 reflecting the worst. This suggests that quality of life is multidimensional. The QoLi has been used to generate an indication of the quality of life of cancer patients and patients with chronic disease. Doctors or other assessors of patients have used the QoLi questionnaire on their clients. There is also a version of the QoLi that can be used in patient self-assessment. More generally, the QoLi has been used in healthcare systems in Canada, the US, France, Germany and Australia. *See* **Health gain; Health index; Health profile; Health status; Index number; Index of health-related quality of life; QALY; Quality of life**.

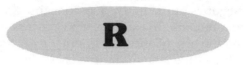

Ramsey pricing principle of public finance
The notion that goods and services with the lowest degrees of responsiveness to price changes should be taxed more heavily to raise tax revenue. Examples include tobacco and petrol. *See* **Consumer's surplus; Elasticity; Own price elasticity of demand; Own price elasticity of supply; Producer's surplus**.

Randomised control trial
A trial to determine the relative merits of interventions in which patients are randomly assigned to one of the possible interventions. For example, in a study patients may be randomised to receive a placebo or a new anti-ulcer medicine. *See* **Gold standard; Placebo; Systematic review**.

Rate of return regulation
A method of controlling how much reward one can retain from sales. For example, the UK government regulates pharmaceutical companies' rates of return on capital employed on sales of medicines to the UK's National Health Service under the pharmaceutical price regulation scheme (PPRS). Under the 1993–98 PPRS agreement, pharmaceutical companies could generally retain between 17% and 21% return on capital employed on sales of medicines to the NHS. *See* **Pharmaceutical price regulation scheme; Price cap regulation; Reduced-form regulation; Reference pricing; Regulation; Theory of second best**.

Rational expectations
A theory of how people make decisions. It is a school of thought in economics that believes that people do not make systematic errors in their decision making or when they are making predictions. Thus, any errors that do occur are purely random. A strong version of rational expectations is that people have perfect foresight, perfect knowledge and understanding of how the economy works, full information, instant and complete

learning capabilities. A weaker version of rational expectations is that people act *as if* they have these characteristics.

Mathematically, rational expectations can be expressed as follows:

$$E_{t-i} = A_t$$

Where, in general terms, E_{t-i} is your expectations of the event at time $_{t-i}$ and A_t is what actually happens at time $_t$. Notice if $_i$ is zero, this means that what happens today is what you expected to happen. *See* **Adaptive expectations**.

Rationing
A method of allocating resources. It is neither new nor unique to healthcare systems. The word 'rationing' brings out many emotions and generates much debate. With respect to patients, it is a method of deciding who gets what treatment, where, when and how.

The underlying need for rationing is that the healthcare system cannot do everything for everyone in need and therefore choices have to be made. Yet it is not just a question of funding, because even if there was enough funding for all healthcare needs to be met, this may not be an efficient use of the economy's resources as there is an opportunity cost involved in every decision. For example, the economy may be better off if some of the funds went into education, social care or transport improvements, rather than healthcare.

The controversies surrounding the term 'rationing' stem from the fact that there are many ways of making choices, various issues on what information is used, question marks about the distribution of gains and losses, equity and differences in perspectives. Rationing decisions are a fusion of subjective and objective reasoning.

Various ways of rationing in healthcare include: the use of waiting lists; according to the potential for health improvements; according to the greatest clinical need; according to the cheapest operations being performed first; according to government targets; according to ability to pay; according to willingness to pay; by priorities established by asking the population; according to clinicians' priorities; according to age; according to gender; according to the type of adverse medical condition; by insurance risk or insurance coverage. *See* **Opportunity cost; Paradox of voting; Priority setting**.

Reduced-form regulation
Occurs when regulation cannot capture all eventualities or factors. There is a limit to the scope of regulation and it is impossible to regulate for all

eventualities using all possible instruments of regulation all the time. There-fore, it follows that regulation is neither complete nor comprehensive. Reduced-form regulation is the norm. *See* **Regulation**.

Reference pricing

A technique of paying or setting the price of a healthcare product with reference to prices of products in the class of healthcare goods or services.

For example, suppose there are currently five anti-cholinesterase medicines used for patients with neuromuscular disorders. Suppose the medicines cost £1.50, £2, £3.75, £4.30 and £5.15 per defined daily dose. If the primary care group manager uses a simple reference price system on the basis of average costs, the group would pay £3.34 for any medicine (£1.50 + £2 + £3.75 + £4.30 + £5.15)/5. Notice here that the group pays a price above the cheapest two medicines and below the other three.

Another type of internal reference price system is to pay the second lowest price for any of the medicines (£2 in the above example) or to pay the median price for any of the medicines (£3.75 in the above example).

In pharmaceuticals, reference pricing can be internal (as in Germany since 1989, the Netherlands since 1991 and Denmark since 1993) whereby the price the healthcare purchasers pay is determined by the price of similar therapeutic or pharmacological pharmaceuticals available in the country. Alternatively, reference pricing can be external (as in Portugal and Eire since 1990) whereby the price paid for medicines reflects the price of the product in other countries. Portugal's reference basket includes France, Italy and Spain whereas Eire's reference basket includes the UK, Germany, Denmark, France and the Netherlands. Reference pricing can be weighted by volume or calculated by converting the prescribed volume of medication into defined daily doses (DDDs) as above. Sometimes called yardstick pricing. *See* **DDD; Pharmaceutical price regulation scheme; Price cap regulation; Rate of return regulation; Reduced-form regulation; Regulation; Yardstick pricing**.

Reagan's Executive Order 12291

Although Presidents Nixon, Ford and Carter all tried to use economics to help improve decision making, it was not until the time of President Reagan that more formal requirements of assessment of policy came about in the US. Under Order 12291 of 1981, it became a mandatory requirement for US regulatory agencies to use a type of economic assessment when the agency was proposing new regulations, proposing amendments to existing regulations or developing legislation affecting regulations. Under Order

12291 the regulatory agencies had to provide economic evidence, in the guise of a dossier called the regulatory impact analysis (RIA), to the Office of Management and Budget for consideration in taking the agency's proposal through government. *See* **Compliance cost assessment; Regulatory impact analysis.**

Regressive tax
Exists when the tax paid as a proportion of, say, income is higher the lower one's income. *See* **Progressive tax; Proportional tax.**

Regulation
No universal definition of what regulation means actually exists. If we regulate a clock we are usually aiming to have the clock do precisely what it is supposed to do: tell the correct time. Other definitions of regulation include: rules set (by law) to determine how exchange is to take place; rules defining conditions about the way in which exchange (buyer–seller) is conducted; predetermined rules which create the framework to ensure relatively free and fair market behaviour; directives or requirements with sanctions for non-compliance; rules and agencies to set the number of purchasers and providers, their relationships to each other and to other parties.

A more germane definition of regulation is as follows: regulation is the act of controlling and conditioning markets and market behaviour. The controls can affect the structure, conduct, incentives, performance or rewards in markets.

This definition is flexible enough to allow for non-governmental bodies to be seen as regulators, e.g. the General Medical Council in the UK regulates the practices of UK doctors. *See* **Reduced-form regulation; Regulatory impact analysis.**

Regulatory impact analysis
A technique for determining the consequences of a regulation or set of regulations. Each regulatory impact analysis (RIA) has to contain the following:

1 A description of the potential costs of the regulation including any adverse effects that could not be quantified in monetary terms.

2 An indication of those parties that would bear the costs.

3 A description of the potential benefits of the regulation, including any beneficial effects that could not be quantified in monetary terms.

4 An indication of those parties that would obtain these benefits.

5 An indication of the potential net benefits of the regulation including an evaluation of effects not quantified in money terms.

6 A description of alternative approaches that could substantially achieve the same regulatory goal(s) at lower cost.

7 An analysis of the potential benefits and costs of the alternatives.

8 A brief explanation of why such alternatives, if proposed, could not be adopted.

9 Unless covered by the point immediately above, an explanation of any legal reasons why the regulation cannot be based on cost–benefit analysis.

Therefore the RIA is concerned with:

- a spatial aspect, i.e. *who* would get *what*;

- a temporal dimension, *when*;

- an impact or distribution dimension on *how* the parties identified would get the costs and benefits; and

- an opportunity cost consideration.

See **British Medical Journal guidelines for economic evaluations; Compliance cost assessment; Cost–benefit analysis; Cost-effectiveness analysis; Cost-minimisation analysis; Cost–utility analysis; Economic assessment decision tree; Guidance on Good Practice in the Conduct of Economic Evaluations of Medicines; Opportunity cost; Reagan's Executive Order 12291.**

Relative poverty
A situation of destitution, penury or privation with respect to a particular benchmark of well-being. Sometimes the benchmark is the average standard of living in the country. Anyone living below the average would be classified as living in relative poverty. *See* **Absolute poverty.**

Relative risk

The ratio of the incidence of an event in the group of people undergoing a new care regime or exposed to a risk, compared to the incidence of the event in the group of people in usual care or not exposed to the risk. The 'event' or outcome could be death or disease, e.g. stroke, fractured neck of femur.

Table 19 Relative risk

| | Outcome | | | |
	Event occurs	Event does not occur	Total	Risk of events
New care or exposure	a (1)	b (2)	a + b = 3	X = a/(a + b) = 1/3
Usual care or not exposed	c (3)	d (4)	c + d = 7	Y = c/(c + d) = 3/7
Totals	a + c = 4	b + d = 6	a + b + c + d = 10	

Using Table 19, mathematically, the relative risk (RR) is calculated as follows:

$$RR = \frac{a/(a+b)}{c/(c+d)} = \frac{X}{Y}$$

Using the data in Table 19 as an example, then:

$$RR = \frac{1/(1+2)}{3/(3+4)} = \frac{1/3}{3/7} = 0.78$$

If RR = 1, then the risk of the event (e.g. developing the disease) is the same in both groups. If RR < 1, then the risk of the event is less in the new care or exposed group compared to the other group. An example could be a lower risk of fractured neck of femur by preventive medication in the new care regime.

If RR > 1, then the risk of the event is greater for those in the new care or exposed group compared to the other group. See **Absolute risk; Absolute risk reduction; Likelihood ratio; Odds; Odds ratio; Relative risk reduction**.

Relative risk reduction

A measure of percentage reduction of events in one regime compared to another.

Suppose in a special care baby unit, 9.6% of babies die under standard care but 2.4% would die under a new care regime. Then the relative risk reduction (RRR) is calculated as follows:

$$RRR = \frac{9.6 - 2.4}{9.6} = 0.75$$

So the new care regime would reduce the risk of death by 75% compared to the usual care regime.

In terms, the RRR can be written as:

$$RRR = \frac{\text{Events in usual care} - \text{Events in new regime}}{\text{Events in usual care}}$$

As another example, we can look at the RRR in terms of comparing outcomes from different care regimes or exposure.

Table 20 Relative risk reduction

	Outcome			
	Event occurs	Event does not occur	Total	Risk of events
New care or exposure	a (1)	b (2)	a + b = 3	X = a/(a + b) = 1/3
Usual care or not exposed	c (3)	d (4)	c + d = 7	Y = c/(c + d) = 3/7
Totals	a + c = 4	b + d = 6	a + b + c + d = 10	

Using Table 20, mathematically, the RRR can be written as:

$$RRR = 1 - X/Y = (Y - X)/Y$$

We can illustrate this by looking at a set of hypothetical data in Table 20:

$$RRR = (3/7 - 1/3)/(3/7) = 0.29$$

which implies that the new care regime lowers the risk of the event by 29% compared to usual care. *See* **Absolute risk; Absolute risk reduction; Incidence; Likelihood ratio; Number needed to treat; Odds; Odds ratio; Relative risk**.

Revealed preference
A person's disclosure of their preference amongst options. For example, a patient with advanced-stage leukaemia may reveal that she would prefer to die at home rather than in an institution. *See* **Conjoint analysis; Decision tree; Standard gamble; Time trade-off**.

Risk averse
A person is said to be risk averse if they are disinclined, opposed and reluctant to do something that involves a risk. For example, a risk-averse person will refuse to play a game even where they have a 50/50 chance of winning, i.e. a mathematically fair game. *See* **Risk neutral; Risk seeker**.

Risk neutral
A person is said to be risk neutral if they are indifferent to risk. *See* **Risk averse; Risk seeker**.

Risk seeker
A person is said to be a risk seeker if they pursue risk: they take decisions even when the odds are against them. *See* **Risk averse; Risk neutral**.

Rosenthal outcome
Occurs when an examiner finds what they *a-priori* expected to find in the examination. It can occur in at least three ways:

1 it may just be that they correctly and fully specified the hypothesis;

2 it may just be serendipitous;

3 it may be that the data or method of analysis was designed to precondition the results.

See **Outcome; Systematic review**.

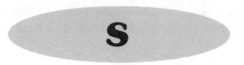

S

Scarcity

A shortage with respect to the amount of demand. If something is not in demand then, even if it is rare, it is not scarce in economic terms. The existence of scarcity is one of the main reasons for the existence of the discipline of economics. *See* **Opportunity cost.**

Sellers' market

Exists when there is more demand for the healthcare product than available supply. This suggests that the sellers have the upper hand in the market and can expect to secure higher prices, offer lower quality or volume for the same price. *See* **Buyers' market; Equilibrium; Excess demand.**

Semifixed costs

Occur when, up to a point, costs do not rise as output rises but after that point, costs do rise. *See* **Cost (form of cost); Fixed cost; Variable cost.**

Sensitivity

The proportion of positive test results in people with the disease. In Table 21 the sensitivity (SEN) is calculated as follows:

$$SEN = a/(a + c)$$

Using the numbers in Table 21 as an illustration:

$$SEN = 10/(10 + 30) = 0.25$$

Sometimes called the true-positive rate.

Table 21 Sensitivity

	True condition of the person tested		
Test result	Has the adverse medical condition	Does not have the adverse medical condition	Total
Positive	a (10)	b (20)	a + b (30)
Negative	c (30)	d (40)	c + d (70)
Total	a + c (40)	b + d (60)	a + b + c + d (100)

See **Specificity; True-positive rate**.

Sensitivity analysis

Methods of calculating how responsive results are to changes in the under-lying variables or assumptions. The following example comes from Coventry Health Authority. Suppose a community care system is put in place to avoid inappropriate hospital admissions. By having a district nurse assess the patient and ensuring that the patient gets what they need, this may avoid inappropriate hospital admissions. However, it is not clear exactly what would have happened to the patient if the district nurse service was not in place. Therefore we may wish to determine how sensitive any savings from avoiding inappropriate hospital admission are by changing the underlying parameters of:

- what the patient would have cost had they gone into hospital (cost);

- how many of the patients would have gone into hospital in absence of the service (volume).

See **Multiple parameter sensitivity analysis; Needs assessment; Single parameter sensitivity analysis; Threshold point analysis**.

Short-Form 36

A measure of a person's general health based on responses to 36 questions. The Short-Form 36 questionnaire (SF-36) covers eight areas (Table 22).

Table 22 SF-36

1 Bodily pain
2 General health perception
3 Mental health (psychological distress and well-being)
4 Physical functioning
5 Role limitation due to emotional problems
6 Role limitation due to physical health
7 Social functioning
8 Vitality

From the answers to the 36 questions, a score is assigned to each of the eight areas and the higher the scores, the greater the well-being of the person. *See* **EuroQol; Health measurement pyramid; Health profile; Health status; Index of health-related quality of life; QALY; Quality of life; Nottingham Health Profile; Sickness Impact Profile.**

Short-run
The time period in which most inputs cannot be varied. *See* **Long-run.**

Sickness Impact Profile
A health status measurement instrument designed to capture the impact of sickness on a person's well-being. It is a general measure of health status and is neither disease nor population specific. The Sickness Impact Profile (SIP) consists of 136 items and has, for example, been used in patients with chronic heart disease. There are 11 dimensions of health in the profile (Table 23).

Table 23 Dimensions of the Sickness Impact Profile

1 Alertness behaviour
2 Ambulation
3 Body care and movement
4 Communication
5 Eating
6 Emotional behaviour
7 Home management
8 Mobility
9 Recreation and pastimes
10 Sleep and rest
11 Social interaction and work

The collection of answers to the SIP can be used to signal the well-being of the patient and how their sickness affects them. It can also be used to elicit people's values of certain healthcare states.

Attempts have been made to turn the SIP, which is a profile, into a health index by weighing the answers from 0 to 100 (with greater results meaning greater impairment) and adding the figures to reveal a single number. The main problems in such an exercise are: who decides what the weight should be and are the results additive? *See* **EuroQol; Health gain; Health measurement pyramid; Health profile; Health status; Index of health-related quality of life; Nottingham Health Profile; Quality of life.**

Single parameter sensitivity analysis
Techniques of calculating how responsive results are to changes in one parameter or assumption. Figure 36 shows single parameter sensitivity analysis when the quantity of medicines bought by a primary care group to treat patients with prostate cancer changes. *See* **Multiple parameter sensitivity analysis; Sensitivity analysis.**

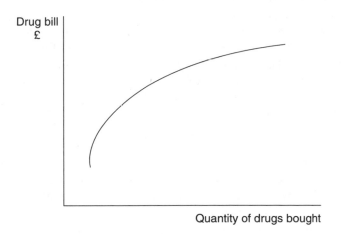

Figure 36 Single parameter sensitivity analysis

Slutsky decomposition
Teases out two effects on demand from a change in the price of the product: the income effect and the substitution effect (Figure 37).

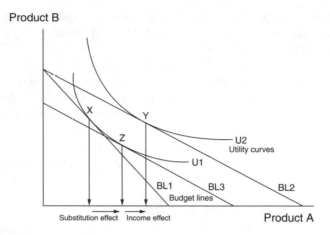

Figure 37 Slutsky decomposition: income effect and substitution effect

The income effect is the change in demand for a healthcare product due to a change in real income when the price of a healthcare product changes. The substitution effect is the change in demand for a healthcare product due to a change in relative prices.

The income effect need not be of the same magnitude or even in the same direction as the substitution effect. The net effect of a price change is found by adding the income effect to the substitution effect. The net effect on demand resulting from a price change can be to lower demand (negative net effect), no change in demand (neutral) or increase demand (positive). *See* **Income effect; Substitution effect**.

Social benefit
The gains to society as a whole from a particular event. *See* **Analytic perspective; Externalities; Pigovian subsidy; Pigovian tax; Social cost**.

Social cost
The cost to society as a whole from a particular event. *See* **Analytic perspective; Externalities; Pigovian subsidy; Pigovian tax; Social benefit**.

Social welfare function
A mathematical relationship which is said to reflect the factors that affect society's well-being. *See* **Welfare**.

Specificity

The proportion of negative test results in people without the disease. In Table 24, the specificity of the test is:

$$SPEC = d/(b + d)$$

Using the numbers as an example:

$$SPEC = 40/(20 + 40) = 0.66$$

Sometimes called the true-negative rate.

Table 24 Specificity

Test result	True condition of the person tested		Total
	Has the adverse medical condition	Does not have the adverse medical condition	
Positive	a (10)	b (20)	a + b (30)
Negative	c (30)	d (40)	c + d (70)
Total	a + c (40)	b + d (60)	a + b + c + d (100)

See **Sensitivity; True-negative rate.**

Specific quality of life measurement instruments

Devices for identifying, recording and measuring distinct aspects of a person's quality of life. *See* **EuroQol; Health measurement pyramid; Health status; Index of health-related quality of life; Nottingham Health Profile; Quality of life; Short-Form 36; Sickness Impact Profile.**

Standard gamble

A technique for eliciting people's value of life and health status. Figure 38 shows a typical standard gamble. Suppose you are in health state A and you can remain as you are or take the following gamble: have a healthcare intervention which will either give you perfect health, with probability Y, or will kill you, with probability 1–Y. The standard gamble can be displayed in a decision tree as seen in Figure 38.

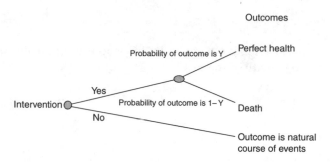

Figure 38 Standard gamble

When the gamble has been carried out once, say hypothetically, the Y is varied until the person becomes indifferent between staying as they are or taking the gamble. This Y is then said to reflect the person's individual preferences and values concerning their quality of life. Sometimes called von Neumann–Morgensten standard gamble. *See* **Conjoint analysis; Decision tree; Revealed preference; Time trade-off; von Neumann–Morgensten standard gamble.**

STAR-PU

An acronym for Specific Therapeutic group, Age, sex, Related Prescribing Unit. It is a method of adjusting prescribing data to reflect the age and sex profile of the patients in each therapeutic group. For example, the cost of endocrine medication is higher for female than for male patients; elderly patients receive more medicines for Parkinson's disease, renal failure and osteoarthritis than other age groups. STAR-PUs reflect an attempt to make more meaningful comparisons of prescribing data over time or between organisations. *See* **ASTRO-PU; DDD; General Practice Research Database; PACT.**

State preference model

A framework which is used to capture different possible states amongst which a person must choose. The model includes details of the states and outcomes and probabilities of achieving the outcomes. *See* **Conjoint analysis; Decision tree; Standard gamble; Time trade-off.**

Statistical significance
If a result is said to be statistically significant at the 5% level, say, this means that we are 95% certain the result did not occur by chance.

Stochastic frontier analysis
Statistical techniques that aim to establish how far a person or organisation is from their optimal level of performance. *See* **Production possibility frontier**.

Straight-line depreciation
Occurs when the rate of depreciation of an asset is constant over time. It can be calculated when information on the initial cost, residual value and life expectancy of the asset is known. The straight-line depreciation (SLD) formula is as follows:

$$SLD = \frac{\text{Initial cost} - \text{Residual value}}{\text{Years of useful working life}}$$

If any three of the factors are known, e.g. SLD, initial cost, years of useful working life, the fourth (in this case residual value) can be determined by rearranging the formula, inserting the known data and working out the result of the fourth component.

For example, if a magnetic resonance imaging (MRI) machine has an expected useful working life of ten years, initially cost £1m and has a residual value at the end of ten years of £50 000 then, on a straight-line depreciation, the calculation is as follows:

$$SLD = \frac{£1\ 000\ 000 - £50\ 000}{10} = £95\ 000$$

which means the MRI depreciates by £95 000 in each of its ten years of useful life.

Figure 39 shows the difference between straight-line depreciation and the declining balance technique (i.e. the declining depreciation rate). *See* **Declining balance technique; Discounting**.

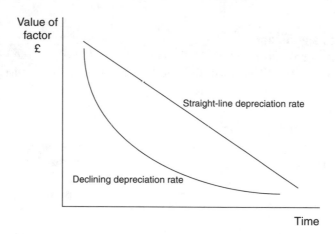

Figure 39 Depreciation

Substitutes
Goods or services are said to be substitutes if the demand for one rises as the price of another rises. For example, the demand for non-laser cataract operations may rise if the price of PHACO laser treatment for cataracts goes up. *See* **Cross price elasticity of demand; Substitution effect**.

Substitution effect
When the price of a product changes, there are two effects: the substitution effect and the income effect. The substitution effect is the change in demand for a healthcare product due to a change in relative prices. Figure 40 gives an illustration of the substitution effect, where the consumer can buy product A and B.

If someone is buying medicine A and other goods and services categorised as B, then with budget line BL1 the best they can do is reach utility U1, at point X. If the price of medicine A falls then, *ceteris paribus*, the budget line moves out to BL2. With this new budget line the person can buy more of medicine A and at least the same amount of the other goods and services B. The person then, at best, reaches utility U2, point Y, where the new budget line, BL2, is tangential to the new utility curve, U2.

The substitution effect is found by rotating the old budget line around the old utility curve U1 until the old budget line, BL1, is parallel to the new budget line, BL2. In Figure 40, this happens when BL1 rotates around to become BL3. The budget line, BL3, is tangential to the utility curve, U1,

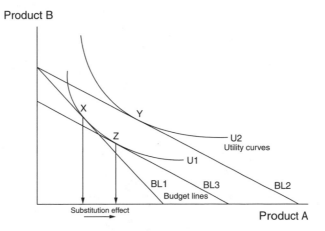

Figure 40 The substitution effect

at point Z. The substitution effect then is measured along the horizontal axis from X of product A to Z of product A.

The substitution effect need not be of the same magnitude or even in the same direction as the income effect. The net effect of a price change is found by adding the income effect to the substitution effect. The net effect on demand resulting from a price change can be to lower demand (negative net effect), no change in demand (neutral) or increase demand (positive). *See* **Income effect**; **Slutsky decomposition**.

Supplier-induced demand

Supplier-induced demand (SID) is said to exist when the supply of a product creates a demand for it. Suppose a hospital buys a new magnetic resonance imaging machine. The hospital staff will wish to see the machine put to use and will therefore indicate to potential purchasers in primary care groups and private health insurers the availability of the machine and concomitant service. Supplier-induced demand is not necessarily an inefficient use of resources.

Supply curve

A locus of quantities of healthcare goods and services that will be provided at different possible prices. Figure 41 shows a normal supply curve (where price is directly related to quantity supplied).

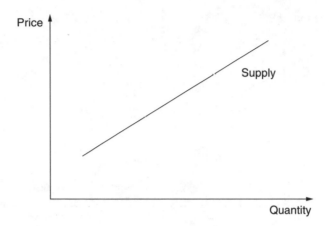

Figure 41 Normal supply curve

Figure 42 shows a backward bending supply curve, with quantity of time at work on the horizontal axis and income on the vertical axis. The supply curve is backward bending to reflect the idea that, initially, as more income is offered, the person does more hours of work but after a point (Ib), a higher income induces fewer hours of work.

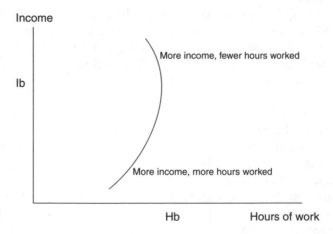

Figure 42 Backward bending supply curve

A distinction has to be made between shifts *in* (*along*) the supply curve (which can be caused by increases in the market price) and shifts *of* the supply curve (which can be caused by changes in technology, factor costs, number of suppliers or market regulations). *See* **Demand curve;**

Giffen good or service; Merit good or service; Normal good or service; Producer's surplus; Public good or service; Supplier-induced demand.

Surrogate endpoints

Sometimes called proxy endpoints, are observation markers that are believed to relate to the primary endpoints of interest. They can be clinical, physiological, chemical or biological identifiers. For example, bone mineral density may be used as a surrogate endpoint for fractured neck of femur; cholesterol levels for cardiovascular mortality; lipid levels for arteriosclerosis; relapse time in multiple sclerosis; cancer cell growth for survival time; viral load in HIV patients. *See* **Outcome**.

Systematic review

An approach to capturing and assessing the evidence by some systematic method, where all the components of the approach and the assessment are made explicit and documented.

Some examples of components include: the research question being addressed; publication entry and exit selection criteria; areas where evidence was looked for (e.g. electronic databases such as Medline); the methods used in the evidence; how the results were collated; how the key messages were derived.

Systematic reviews can be based on several premises:

1 Large quantities of information must be made into palatable pieces for consumption.

2 Such reviews integrate critical pieces of available information.

3 A review is usually quicker and less expensive than a new study.

4 The generalisability of the evidence can be established.

5 The consistency of relationships can be established.

6 Inconsistencies in the evidence can be determined.

7 Gaps in the evidence can be identified.

8 Increases in the statistical power of studies can be achieved.

See **Accountability; Due process; Duhem's irrefutability theory; Falsificationism; Grey literature; Lakatosian hard-core, protective belt; National Institute of Clinical Excellence; Transitivity; Transparency.**

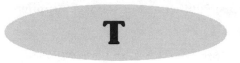

T

Take-up rate

The number of people taking up a service compared to the total number eligible to take up the service. Suppose, in a health action zone, 1000 women in their menopause are eligible for cancer screening but, for various reasons, only 850 have the screening. Then, the take-up rate is 0.85 (850/1000).

Estimates of the take-up rate of a service are important for assisting planning, priority setting, financial viability and resource allocation. Reasons for a low take-up rate could be: ignorance of the availability of the service; lack of access to the service; poor quality of the service or aftercare (real or perceived); a reluctance to use the service if there are no satisfactory means of redress if something goes wrong; side effects of possible treatment; fear of having to deal with the news of having the disease. *See* **Demand**; **Health action zone**; **Health improvement programme**; **Need**; **Supply**.

Tax avoidance

A set of legal techniques that aim to reduce the amount of tax paid by a person or organisation. *See* **Tax evasion**.

Tax evasion

A set of illegal techniques that aim to reduce the amount of tax paid by a person or organisation. *See* **Tax avoidance**.

Technical efficiency

Occurs when maximum output is achieved with minimum inputs. *See* **Allocative efficiency**; **Efficiency**.

Terms of trade

The index of export prices divided by the index of import prices. *See* **Index number**; **Purchasing power parity**.

Theory of second best

The theory of second best states that when it is impossible to have all conditions necessary for a first-best solution, the second-best solution may be where none of the other conditions are met. Thus, if six criteria are needed for the first-best state and one, say perfect information on the therapeutic effects of a medication, is not met, this does not imply that the other five criteria have to be met to achieve the second-best state. Indeed, the second-best state may be where none of the six criteria exist even if criteria 1, 2, 3, 4 or 5 can be met.

For a first-best state, price will equal marginal cost in each and every activity; this ensures that no one who values a product more than it costs society to produce will be deterred from buying or receiving it. But where price differs from marginal cost in one activity, the second-best state need not be where all other prices equate to their respective marginal costs. *See* **Effectiveness; Efficacy; Efficiency; Marginal cost.**

Third-party payment

Occurs when neither the doctor nor the patient pays the bill for the healthcare that the patient receives. It may be that the patient's health insurer pays the bill, it could be a charity or it could be financed out of general taxation. *See* **Third-party payment problem.**

Third-party payment problem

Occurs when the doctor and patient are insulated, to a degree, from the costs of their decisions as a third party pays the bill. Therefore, the doctor and patient have less incentive to account for the costs of care chosen. *See* **Adverse selection; Moral hazard; Third-party payment; User charges.**

Threshold point analysis

A special case of sensitivity analysis. In commerce, for example, a threshold point is the point at which the organisation makes neither a loss nor a profit. In consumer behaviour, a threshold point is the point at which the consumer is indifferent between the options available. *See* **Break-even diagram; Indifference curve; Profit; Sensitivity analysis.**

Time preference

When people would prefer to choose benefits sooner rather than later and defer costs, they exhibit time preference. *See* **Time trade-off.**

Time trade-off

A technique for estimating a person's value of life. The person is given a choice of living in health state A for ten years or having a healthcare intervention that will improve their health status but reduce their life expectancy. The person is then asked to trade-off the time between living in health state A for ten years or living in a better health state for X number of years. Figure 43 gives an example.

X is varied until the person is indifferent between the options available. *See* **Health status; Indifference curve; Standard gamble**.

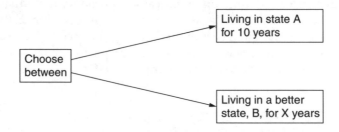

Figure 43 Time trade-off

Total costs

The sum of all costs.

Townsend's index of deprivation

A single number which is said to represent the degree of deprivation of people in a community. The index is made up of the following components:

1 unemployed residents over 16 years of age as a proportion of all economically active residents over 16 years of age in the community;

2 the number of households with one or more persons per room as a proportion of all households in the community;

3 the number of households with no car as a proportion of all households in the community;

4 the number of households not owning their own home as a proportion of all households in the community.

The calculation of the Townsend's index of deprivation is as follows. First, calculate the components individually (e.g. by census survey). Second, take the natural logarithm of components 1 and 2 (not 3 or 4, notice). Third, calculate the Z-scores of the logarithms of elements 1 and 2 and the Z-scores of components 3 and 4. Fourth, apply equal weights to the resulting data. Fifth, add up the numbers to reveal a single index number, which is the Townsend's index of deprivation. The greater the index number, the greater the deprivation. Debate exists on the merits of the components used and the method of calculation employed. *See* **Absolute poverty; Carstair's index of deprivation; Department of Employment index for planning; Index number; Jarman's index of deprivation; Relative poverty.**

Trade-off

Occurs when a choice is made between two seemingly incompatible options. For example, it has been said that there is a trade-off between equity and efficiency in healthcare. *See* **Efficiency; Equity; Equity–efficiency trade-off; Opportunity cost; Time trade-off.**

Transfer earnings

Is the amount of money that a person could earn in their best alternative employment. For example, suppose a university lecturer specialises in finance but could alternatively take a job as Director of Finance in one of the new primary care groups (PCG). If the lecturer could earn £65 000 a year as Director of Finance of the PCG, then that is the amount of their transfer earning. *See* **Economic rent; Opportunity cost.**

Transfer payment

A payment from one group in society to another without any product being produced. Examples include taxation to fund Social Services and unemployment benefit.

Transitivity

A rule in logic whereby more than two factors are ranked. Suppose clinical trials show that the efficacy of medicine A is greater than that of medicine B and the efficacy of medicine B is greater than that of medicine C. If the transitivity law applies, it follows that the efficacy of medicine A must be greater than that of medicine C. When the law applies, it can reduce the number of clinical trials and economic evaluations required to show the relative merits of different medicines. *See* **Systematic review**.

Transparency

Another term for clarity. For example, transparency may relate to a course of action, a decision, a method of analysis or the source of a piece of evidence. *See* **Accountability; Due process; Governance; Systematic review**.

True-negative rate

The proportion of negative test results in people without the disease.

Table 25 True-negative rate

| Test result | True condition of the person tested | | Total |
	Has the adverse medical condition	Does not have the adverse medical condition	
Positive	a (10)	b (20)	a + b (30)
Negative	c (30)	d (40)	c + d (70)
Total	a + c (40)	b + d (60)	a + b + c + d (100)

Using Table 25, the true-negative rate (TNR) is written as follows:

$$TNR = d/(b+d)$$

Using the numbers in Table 25 as an example:

$$TNR = 40/(20 + 40) = 0.66$$

The true-negative rate is another term for specificity. *See* **False-negative rate; False-positive rate; Specificity; True-positive rate**.

True-positive rate

The proportion of positive test results in people with the disease. Mathematically, the true-positive rate (TPR) is written as follows:

$$TPR = a/(a + c)$$

Using the numbers in Table 25 as an illustration:

$$TPR = 10/(10 + 30) = 0.25$$

Sometimes the true-positive rate is called the sensitivity. *See* **False-negative rate; False-positive rate; Sensitivity; True-negative rate.**

Type I error

Occurs when the null hypothesis is wrongly rejected. For example, if one concludes there is a relationship between factors under study when in reality that relationship does not exist. Type I errors, if not corrected, lead to inappropriate use of resources. For example, if someone is diagnosed as having an adverse medical condition then they will usually be given a course of treatment or surgery. In the case of cancer, that treatment could have irreversible physical and psychological effects such as the removal of a breast. If a type I error is made then the patient is having the treatment when in fact they do not have the adverse medical condition. *See* **Type II error.**

Type II error

Occurs when the null hypothesis is wrongly accepted. For example, if one concludes there is no relationship between factors under study, as specified in the null hypothesis, when in reality the relationship exists. Type II errors, if not corrected, lead to inappropriate use of resources. If someone is diagnosed as not having an adverse medical condition then they will not usually be given a course of treatment or surgery. In time, their condition can worsen and, once identified, it may be too late to save the patient or the costs of trying to do so may be substantial. *See* **Type I error.**

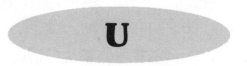

Unemployment

Occurs when a person who would otherwise be working is without a job. It may or may not be voluntary. *See* **Unemployment benefit**.

Unemployment benefit

The welfare payments that a registered unemployed person is entitled to receive. *See* **Take-up rate; Unemployment; Unemployment trap**.

Unemployment trap

Occurs when a person is, or would be, better off registering unemployed, receiving unemployment and welfare benefit, than being in work. *See* **Poverty trap; Unemployment; Unemployment benefit**.

Unit cost

The expense involved in producing one unit. Sometimes called average cost. *See* **Average cost; Cost (form of cost)**.

User charges

Sums of money paid to a healthcare provider for a product. The most common, though certainly not the most popular, is the prescription charge that many people have to pay for NHS-prescribed medicines in the UK. This user charge exists even though one of the founding, and still claimed, principles of the NHS is that it will provide healthcare goods and services free at the point of consumption.

User charges have a variety of effects. They can reduce what are thought to be wasteful or frivolous demands on a service. On the other hand, they can affect legitimate demands on a service because if the patient cannot afford the charge and they have no third party to pay on their behalf, then the existence of the charge will deter use even when they need the health-care product. Table 26 shows the UK's NHS prescription user charges since

1979. The user charges can also act as a means of income generation; the UK's government received around £320m from healthcare user charges in 1996.

Table 26 UK NHS prescription charges since 1979 (per item)

July 1979	£0.45	April 1989	£2.80
April 1980	£0.70	April 1990	£3.05
December 1980	£1.00	April 1991	£3.40
April 1982	£1.30	April 1992	£3.75
April 1983	£1.40	April 1993	£4.25
April 1984	£1.60	April 1994	£4.75
April 1985	£2.00	April 1995	£5.25
April 1986	£2.20	April 1996	£5.50
April 1987	£2.40	April 1997	£5.65
April 1988	£2.60	April 1998	£5.80

See **Copayment**.

Utilitarianism

The idea that the purpose of government is to maximise the utility of the population. It implies that utility can be identified and measured and comparisons can be made between individuals. *See* **Cardinal utility; Ordinal utility**.

Utility

Relates to individual well-being, satisfaction or pleasure. In a publication of 1789, the philosopher Jeremy Bentham defined utility as:

> That property of any object whereby it tends to produce benefit, advantage, pleasure, good or happiness: or to prevent the happening of mischief, pain, evil or unhappiness to the party whose interest is considered.

See **Utility analysis; Utility function; Utils**.

Utility analysis

Techniques of decision making based on the axioms of rational behaviour when a person faces uncertainty. *See* **Conjoint analysis; Cost–utility analysis; Decision tree; Standard gamble; Time trade-off; Utility**.

Utility function

A mathematical formula whereby a person's utility is represented by various factors that can or do affect their utility. *See* **Utility**.

Utility theory

The collection of hypotheses as to what determines a person's utility, whether or not utility is ordinal or cardinal and how to best maximise a person's utility. *See* **Cardinal utility**; **Ordinal utility**; **Utility**; **Utils**.

Utils

Measures of utility. *See* **Utility**.

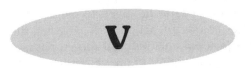

V

Value added

The difference between the selling price of goods and services and the value of the inputs used to produce them. For example, a pharmaceutical company may buy bulk chemicals and turn them into finished medicines for consumption. If inputs are valued at £45m and outputs at £68m then the pharmaceutical company has a value added of £23m.

Value for money table

A table that summarises the relative costs and benefits of one course of action against another (Table 27).

Table 27 Value for money table

Comparing this programme with another			
This course of action	**Costs less**	**Costs the same**	**Costs more**
Provides fewer benefits	4	7	9
Provides the same benefits	2	5	8
Provides greater benefits	I	3	6

Cell 1 is where the course of action would provide more benefits and cost less than the other course of action. Courses of action which would fall into Cells 1, 2, or 3 are generally better value for money.

Cell 9 is where the course of action would provide fewer benefits and actually cost more than the other course of action. Courses of action that would fall into Cells 7, 8, or 9 are generally poorer value for money.

Courses of action that would fall into Cell 5 provide the same benefits at the same costs. For example, this may happen when comparing hospital or home care options for paediatric patients with cystic fibrosis. A decision may be reached on what option to choose based on, say, patient or patient family preferences.

Courses of actions that would fall into Cell 4 cost less but provide fewer benefits. Consideration has to be given to the budgetary implications of implementing this course of action and whether the choice would be acceptable in professional and political terms. Then a decision has to be made by the appropriate authority on whether or not to go for this option.

Courses of action that would fall into Cell 6 cost more and provide greater benefits than the other course of action. In deciding what to do, closer attention has to be paid to the budgetary constraints, i.e. can you afford it, priorities, targets, preferences or clinical guidelines. Then a decision has to be made by the appropriate authority as to whether the course of action would be financially feasible and acceptable in professional and political terms. *See* **Accountability; Due process; Economic assessment decision tree; Priority setting; Programme budgeting; Marginal analysis; Rationing; Systematic review; Transparency.**

Variable costs
Costs that change as volume or activity levels change. *See* **Cost (form of cost); Fixed costs.**

Venn diagram
Is a diagram that shows the extent to which two or more groups have mutually inclusive or mutually exclusive characteristics. Figure 44 presents a Venn diagram of healthcare need, demand and supply. Only in area 5 is there a healthcare need, demand and supply. *See* **Demand; Need; Supply.**

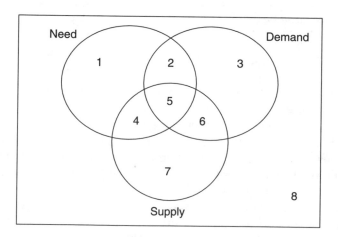

Figure 44 Venn diagram

Vertical equity

The unequal treatment of unequals. *See* **Equity; Horizontal equity**.

Vertical integration

Occurs when one enterprise joins with another that is not at the same stage of production of the product. On the one hand, there may be efficiency gains by reducing transaction costs between the different levels of operation. On the other hand, there is a risk of monopolisation and refusing to supply others at reasonable rates. For example, suppose company A makes base chemicals and B is one of the companies that make medicines from the chemicals. Then if A and B merge the new organisation is AB. AB may change the prices and conditions of the base chemicals that it supplies to others, e.g. companies C and D.

Forward vertical integration happens when an organisation links up with another organisation which is operating further downstream (i.e. nearer the final customer, e.g. patients). For example, a pharmaceutical wholesaler may take over a retail pharmacy.

Backward vertical integration happens when an organisation links up with another organisation further away from the final customer. For example, a pharmaceutical wholesaler may buy a pharmaceutical manufacturer. *See* **Horizontal integration**.

Virement

The movement of funds from one budget heading to another. For example, a doctor may use savings on their medicines budget, as a result of therapeutic or generic substitution, to pay for more expensive medical surgery for some of their other patients. Or, after assessing the primary care group's programme of expenditure and outcomes, the group manager may recommend moving funds from hospital healthcare spending to more community services. Virement may or may not be a legal activity. *See* **Cost centre; Cross subsidisation; Economic rent; Marginal analysis; Profit; Programme budgeting**.

Visual analogue scale

A health status measurement scale in the form of a straight line of defined length, usually 10 cm, anchored at each end by extremes. Respondents are asked to mark a point on the scale that represents their answer to the question set.

For example:

Q1. How would you rate your general health today?

0 ————————————————————————————100

Figure 45 Visual analogue scale: numbers

Some visual analogue scales have numbers at the ends (e.g. as in Figure 45), some have descriptive items (e.g. Figure 46) and some have a combination of descriptors and numbers (e.g. Figure 47). Numerical values are derived by analogue.

| Worst imaginable | . | Best imaginable |
| health state | | health state |

Figure 46 Visual analogue scale: descriptors

0 ————————————————————————————100
Worst imaginable   Best imaginable
health state   health state

Figure 47 Visual analogue scale: numbers and descriptors

Visual analogue scales have been used to measure the quality of life of patients undergoing chemotherapy or radiotherapy. *See* **Guttman Scale; Health gain; Health index; Health measurement pyramid; Index of health-related quality of life; Likert Scale; QALY.**

Volunteer bias
Arises because those who volunteer for a programme may have different characteristics or respond differently to treatment than others. *See* **Hello-goodbye effect**.

von Neumann–Morgensten standard gamble
A technique of eliciting values of health states. For example, a patient is given a choice between an intervention that offers gains in life expectancy

and quality of life but there is also a probability that the patient may be worse off and, indeed, could die as a result of the intervention. Sometimes the technique is used in hypothetical situations to establish patient values of life and interventions. Standard gambles are common in healthcare decision making (e.g. angina, HRT, transplant surgery). *See* **Standard gamble; Time trade-off**.

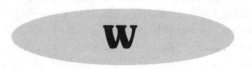

Waiting list
A register of patients who have to wait for the care they are deemed to need. *See* **Demand; Need; Priority setting**.

Welfare
The well-being or prosperity of a person, community or society. *See* **Utility**.

Welfare economics
The study of the social desirability of alternative uses of resources. *See* **Analytic perspective; Welfare**.

Willingness to pay
An amount of money that someone says they would pay for, or do pay for, a healthcare product. It is not the same as ability to pay.

Two ways to establish willingness to pay are: observing and analysing past or current expenditure patterns; asking people directly what they are willing to pay for certain healthcare goods and services.

Both approaches have their strengths and weaknesses. For example, asking someone what they are willing to pay is often a hypothetical scenario and there are difficulties in transferring such responses to real events. If the person asked knows she will not have to pay the full cost anyway, she may suggest a high amount whereas if she knew she would really have to pay the amount, she could suggest a low figure. *See* **Ability to pay; Conjoint analysis; Moral hazard; Third-party payment problem; User charges**.

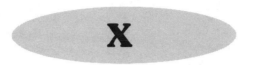

X-inefficiency

Occurs when a person or organisation does not use the resources at their disposal in the most efficient manner. Therefore costs are higher and quality and output lower. *See* **Efficiency; Production possibility frontier; Stochastic frontier analysis**.

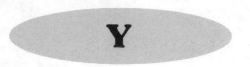

Yardstick pricing

A strategy whereby the prices offered to one party relate to the prices offered to another. For example, a primary care group manager may decide to offer yardstick prices to one hospital based on the prices of similar services from other hospitals. It is sometimes called benchmark pricing. Yardstick pricing may or may not enhance competition. One problem is that the yardstick price offered to one hospital may not relate to the cost of supply from that hospital. *See* **Price cap regulation; Profit; Reduced-form regulation; Reference pricing; Regulation**.

Years of life lost

An indication of the number of years of life lost as a result of premature death. For example, if in one town studies show that bowel cancer kills 100 people five years prematurely, then 500 years of life are lost. *See* **Life expectancy**.

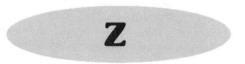

Z-score

Variable values transformed to have a zero mean and unit variance. A Z-score is a type of standardisation used in statistical calculations, e.g. in Jarman's index of deprivation or Townsend's index of deprivation. *See* **Jarman's index of deprivation; Townsend's index of deprivation**.

Zero-based budgeting

A technique of resetting the budget every year to nil and requiring that people or groups provide the evidence to justify any expenditure. *See* **Programme budgeting; Systematic review; Value for money table**.